介入治疗护理
汉英情境对话

Situational Conversation for Nurses
in Interventional Therapy
A Chinese-English Bilingual Handbook

主编　谢明晖　杨继金　陆小英
主审　黄承诚

上海科学技术出版社

图书在版编目（ＣＩＰ）数据

介入治疗护理汉英情境对话 / 谢明晖，杨继金，陆
小英主编. -- 上海：上海科学技术出版社，2024.1
ISBN 978-7-5478-5070-1

Ⅰ．①介… Ⅱ．①谢… ②杨… ③陆… Ⅲ．①介入性
治疗－护理－英语－口语 Ⅳ．①R473

中国版本图书馆CIP数据核字(2021)第143246号

介入治疗护理汉英情境对话

主编　谢明晖　杨继金　陆小英

上海世纪出版(集团)有限公司　出版、发行
上海科学技术出版社
(上海市闵行区号景路 159 弄 A 座 9F - 10F)
邮政编码 201101　　www.sstp.cn
江阴金马印刷有限公司印刷
开本 787×1092　1/40　印张 5
字数：150 千字
2024 年 1 月第 1 版　2024 年 1 月第 1 次印刷
ISBN 978 - 7 - 5478 - 5070 - 1/R·2174
定价：48.00 元

本书如有缺页、错装或坏损等严重质量问题，请向工厂联系调换

内容提要

　　本书以护士对患者的健康教育为核心,聚焦介入科临床护理工作实践,总结了工作中 50 多个常见情境的汉英对话,包括射频消融术、冷冻消融术、微波消融术、粒子植入术、门-体静脉支撑架分流术、载药微球等治疗的宣教,以及检查宣教、药物宣教、并发症宣教、康复宣教、安全宣教等,每个场景分别按专业单词(glossary)、汉英对话(scenario)、短语(phrases)进行阐述。

　　全书提供了介入治疗护理专业英文口语的情境学习指导,实用性强,可帮助护士在学习专业知识的同时提升英语交流能力。

编写人员

主　　编	谢明晖	杨继金	陆小英
副主编	韩文军	曹　洁	李冬梅
主　　审	黄承诚		
参编人员	（按姓氏笔画排序）		

	王　迪	王　菲	王　瑶
	包　蓉	冯晓青	成伟静
	刘　彤	刘丽红	江　薇
	孙　洁	孙佳欢	李　娜
	李梅艳	李淑英	吴　双
	张玉蕾	张婷婷	屈正荣
	赵汉美	胡　娜	施李鹃
	高　阳	凌　芝	储丹凤
	曾春梅	路晨曦	

前　言

随着介入治疗不断取得成效,介入护理学在几代介入治疗领域前辈的不断努力下,也得到了快速发展,并确定了其在临床的重要地位。

现代护理学强调以人为本、以患者为中心的护理模式。在护理工作中,护士和患者交谈疾病的治疗方法、并发症、注意事项及健康教育,优质护理的理念不断深入。护士的入院宣教可协助患者积极调整好心理状态,尽快适应环境,为后期的护患沟通打下基础。患者良好情绪的建立有着非常重要的意义,能减轻护士的工作压力,减少医患纠纷,缓解并发症带给患者的紧张情绪。

本书将介入护理人员平时的工作场景一一呈现,并以汉英对话的形式展现,其中包括日常交流、专科宣教、术后指导等,有通用性,也有专科性。希望介入护理人员通过本书学习,能提升护患教育水平。

笔者编写本书的另一个目的是希望能统一、规范日常用语,以便护患以及护士之间沟通。在编写过程中,我们借鉴了很多护理前辈的经验,将资料进行了系统的归纳和总结。在此,感谢参编此书的医护同仁及给予这本书帮助的老师和朋友。希望此书能对大家有所帮助。限于笔者的水平与能力,书中难免存在不足,敬请广大读者批评指正。

谢明晖

目 录

Interventional Nursing
介入护理

Nursing Care of the Use and Observation of Antineoplastic Drugs
抗肿瘤药物使用与观察的护理

Health Education of Various Types of Catheter Care
各类导管护理的健康教育

Specialized Nursing
专科护理

Health Education for Hospitalized Patients
住院患者的健康教育

Interventional Nursing

介入护理

1. Health Education for Patients with Liver Cancer Before Interventional Therapy
肝癌介入治疗术前患者的健康教育

[Glossary]

interventional surgery	介入手术
postoperative infection	术后感染
minimally invasive surgery	微创手术
limb	肢体
vomit	呕吐
symptom	症状

[Scenario]

护士：您好，我是您的责任护士丽丽，请问您叫什么名字？

N：Good morning/afternoon! My name is Li Li, I am your primary nurse. May I have your name please?

患者：王芳。

P：Wang Fang.

护士：因为您明天要做介入治疗，现在我将告诉您手术前后需要注意的事项。

N：As you know you are going to have an interventional surgery tomorrow, I am going to explain the procedure and some important issues before and after the procedure.

患者：好的。

P：OK, thanks.

护士：您有过食物和药物过敏史吗，如青霉素、碘油？

N：Are you allergic to any food or drugs? such as penicillin or iodized oil?

患者：没有。

P：No.

护士：为降低术后感染风险，请您手术前一天洗澡，换上干净衣服。

N：To reduce the risk of postoperative infection, we advise our patients to take a shower and change clothes the day before the surgery.

患者：好的，没问题。

P：No problem.

护士：您今天晚上8点后除饮水外不要再吃其他任何食物，但之前可以正常饮食；从明天清晨开始禁食、禁水。术前让您禁食的目的是预防术中呕吐。这些我们明天早上还会再次提醒您。

N：In order to prevent vomiting during the surgery, do not eat any food except water after 8 o'clock tonight. You should not have any food or water from tomorrow morning. We'll remind you again by the time.

患者：好的，知道了。

P：I got it.

护士：您在术前需要排空大小便。避免伤口出血，术后需要平卧，术肢制动6小时，12小时后可以下床活动。

N：You need to empty your bowel and bladder before the procedure. After the procedure you have to lie on your back and stay in the bed for 12 hours. During this period, we have to limit your limbs movement for 6 hours to avoid bleeding.

患者：好的。

P：OK.

护士：术后可能会出现疼痛、发热、呕吐等反应，您不要紧张，这是术后正常反应，请及时告知我们，医生会对症处理。

N：Common reactions after the procedure are pain, fever, vomiting and so on. You may experience some of those symptoms. Please let us know any discomforts so we can treat it accordingly.

患者：知道了。

P：I see.

护士：介入治疗是微创手术，手术时间短，您不要紧张，放松情绪。

N：The interventional surgery is a minimally invasive surgery with short operating time. I understand that you might feel nervous. Please try to take it easy.

患者：好的，我之前做过一次治疗。

P：All right, I had one before.

护士：好的，如果您还有什么疑问可以随时问我。

N：Good! Do you have any question?

患者：好的，谢谢。

P：No. Thank you!

护士：谢谢您的配合。

N：Great! Thank you for your cooperation.

[Phrases]

have a surgery	做手术
take a shower	洗澡
change clothes	换衣服
prevent vomiting	预防呕吐
take it easy	别紧张

2. Health Education for Patients with Liver Cancer After Interventional Therapy
肝癌介入治疗术后患者的健康教育

[Glossary]

constipation	便秘
immunity	免疫力
cold	感冒
venous thrombus	静脉血栓

[Scenario]

护士：王芳，您做完介入治疗后有什么不舒服吗？

N：Wang Fang，how are you doing after the surgery？

患者：没有，我什么时候可以下床活动？

P：I am OK. When can I get off my bed？

护士：没有什么不舒服的话，您明天早上就可以下床活动了，要多喝水，多走动，预防下肢静脉血栓形成。

N：You may get off your bed tomorrow morning. In fact，we encourage our patients to do more walking and drink more water to reduce the risk of venous thrombus in the lower limbs.

患者：好的，那我能吃点什么呢？

P：Fine，what kind of food may I eat？

护士：您可以吃一些稀饭、面条、馄饨、蒸蛋等易消化的食物，以及富含纤维素的蔬菜、水果等，以保证大便通畅。如发生便秘，请及时告知医生。

N：Any healthy food you may like. But we recommend some balanced and easily digestible food like porridge，noodles，wonton，steamed eggs and some fresh fruits and vegetables with rich fibers. Some patients may have the problem of constipation, if it happens, please tell the doctor in time.

患者：好的。

P：OK.

护士：术后您的免疫力会有所下降，要注意保暖，保证充足的睡眠，不要着凉、感冒。

N：Your immunity will be influenced. Make sure you have enough sleep and keep warm to prevent a cold.

患者：好的，我会注意的。

P：I see, I will be careful.

护士：术后可能会发热，体温没超过 38.5 ℃，请多饮水，如超过 38.5 ℃请及时告知医生。

N：Having a fever is a common symptom after the surgery. We don't treat it if the temperature is under 38.5 ℃. Just drink more water. But if it's above 38.5 ℃, please inform the doctor.

患者：好的。我什么时候可以洗澡？

P：OK, when can I take a shower?

护士：术后第 2 天就可以洗澡了。

N：The next day after the operation.

患者：知道了，那我回家要注意什么呢？

P：Good, what should I pay attention to when I am at home?

护士：您需要保持乐观情绪，建立积极的生活方式，避免剧烈运动，注意全面摄入营养，戒烟、戒酒。

N：We advise our patients to have an optimistic life attitude, and have a good life style such as moderate excises and healthy diets and avoid the alcohol and smoking.

患者：我会注意的。

P：OK, I will.

护士：请出院后定期随访肝功能、血常规、CT 等检查，按医生的要求定时服用药物。

N：After discharge，please keep your routine follow-up with our doctors，including hepatic function，blood test，CT scan and take the medicine our doctor prescribed regularly.

患者：好的。

P：OK.

护士：如有哪里不舒服，随时打铃叫我，我也会经常过来看您的。

N：You could ring the bell at any time when you feel uncomfortable. We are always here to help.

患者：好的，谢谢。

P：That's great，thank you.

护士：不客气。

N：You are welcome.

[Phrases]

after discharge　　　　　　　　出院后

3. Health Education for Patients in Perioperative Period of Uterine Artery Embolization
子宫动脉栓塞术围手术期患者的健康教育

[Glossary]

uterine	子宫的
artery	动脉
embolization	栓塞
uterine fibroid	子宫肌瘤
trauma	创伤
chronic	慢性的
endometritis	子宫内膜炎
multiple	多次的
pregnancy	怀孕
delivery	生产
estrogen	雌激素
gynecological	妇科的
degeneration	退化;恶化
leucorrhea	白带
backache	背疼;腰酸
bladder	膀胱
menstruation	月经

[Scenario]

患者：张护士，我有一个问题想要咨询您。

P：Nurse Zhang, I have a question for you.

护士：好的，您有什么疑问？

N：Yes. What can I do for you?

患者：医生说我是子宫肌瘤，到底是怎么引起的？

P：I was told that I have uterine fibroid. Could you

explain to me what causes the uterine fibroid?

护士：子宫肌瘤的确切原因尚不清楚。一般认为,多次妊娠和分娩时子宫壁的创伤和慢性子宫内膜炎可能是导致此病的主要原因。此外,可能还与高雌激素的刺激有关。

N：The exact cause of uterine fibroid is not clear. However it is commonly believed that it is associated with trauma and chronic endometritis during multiple pregnancies and deliveries. It is also associated with the stimulation of high estrogen level.

患者：哦,这样啊! 我是体检时发现的,一般都有哪些症状呢?

P：Oh，I see. Mine was found during the physical examination. What are the common symptoms of this disease?

护士：多数人无明显症状,妇科检查时发现。症状与肌瘤部位、生长速度及肌瘤有无变性有关。一般会有月经改变、白带增多、腰酸、下腹坠胀、腹痛。肌瘤压迫膀胱时,可能会出现尿频、尿潴留等症状。

N：In most people it does not have any obvious symptoms; it is usually an incidental finding in gynecological examinations. The symptoms depend on the location, growth rate and existence of degeneration of the fibroid. The common symptoms include menstrual changes, increasing leucorrhea, backache, abdominal distension and abdominal pain. Frequent urination and urinary retention may occur when the fibroids compress the bladder.

患者：那常规的治疗方法是什么?

P：What are the treatment options?

护士：医生一般会进行子宫动脉栓塞术。

N：In our department we usually treat uterine fibroid with

uterine artery embolization.

患者：谢谢，那我手术要注意一些什么吗？

P：Thank you, what should I pay attention to for the surgery?

护士：这是一个微创治疗，不要担心。治疗前需要禁食、水4 小时，术前可能会根据情况用一些消炎药。现在请在病房等待，医生会在您签手术知情同意书时为您详细讲解的。

N：This is a minimally invasive treatment. Please do not worry about it too much. You need to fast for 4 hours before the surgery and doctors may prescribe some anti-inflammatory medicine after the surgery. Now just stay in your ward. The doctor will explain the details when you sign the informed consent.

患者：术后我需要注意什么？

P：What shall I pay attention to after the surgery?

护士：需要注意个人卫生，保持良好的生活习惯。术后 3个月内禁止性生活、盆浴及剧烈运动，以免泌尿生殖系统感染，有生育需求的 1 年内应避孕。栓塞治疗后，一般 1～3 个月后月经周期、月经量恢复正常。3个月后月经仍不正常，或出现下腹坠痛、阴道出血或异常分泌物、尿频或突发性血尿及大便伴脓血、发热等症状，请及时就诊。如果一切正常，请在术后 3、6、12 个月来院做影像学检查，观察肌瘤的缩小情况和瘤体的密度变化。不知道我说的您都明白了吗？

N：You should pay attention to personal hygiene and maintain a good life style. In general, sex, bathing and strenuous exercises should be avoided for the first 3 months after the surgery to reduce the risk of urinary infection. No pregnancy within 12 months after the surgery by using contraception. Your menstrual cycle and amount will return to normal after one to three months of the surgery. You should come to see the doctor if menstruation is still abnormal three months after the surgery, or when symptoms like lower abdominal pain, vaginal bleeding, abnormal discharge, frequent urination, hematuria or blood in the stool, fever appear. We will schedule your follow-up visits 3, 6 and 12 months after the surgery. During those visits we will do radiological examination of the uterus to check the reduction of fibroid size. Do you have more questions?

患者：明白了，讲解很详细。

P: No. You explained it in great detail.

护士：希望对您有所帮助。出院的时候，我们会发纸质版的出院宣教，您也可以关注康复助手。

N: I hope it is helpful to you. We will give you a pamphlet on discharge education. You can also follow our rehabilitation assistant.

患者：好的。谢谢！我现在没有那么紧张了。

P: All right. Thank you! I'm much relieved now.

护士：不客气。

N: You're welcome.

[**Phrases**]

physical examination	体检
obvious symptom	明显症状
growth rate	生长速度
abdominal distension	腹胀
frequent urination	尿频
anti-inflammatory medicine	消炎药
informed consent	知情同意书

4. Health Education for Patients Before Radiofrequency Ablation
射频消融术前患者的健康教育

［Glossary］

radiofrequency ablation（RFA）	射频消融术
heat	热；加热
normal tissue	正常组织
painkiller	止疼药
sweat	出汗
ultrasound	超声

［Scenario］

护士：您好！请问您是李先生吗？我是您的责任护士王芳。

N：Hello! Are you Mr. Li? I'm your primary nurse, my name is Wang Fang.

患者：我是，你好。

P：Yes, I am. Nice to meet you.

护士：您今天需要做 RFA 治疗。

N：The doctor will perform RFA treatment for you today.

患者：好的。

P：OK.

护士：请问您之前进行过 RFA 治疗吗？

N：Have you ever had any RFA treatment before?

患者：没有。

P：No.

护士：那我现在给您大致讲解一下，好吗？

N：May I give you a brief introduction about it?

患者：好的。

P：Yes, please.

护士：RFA 通过使组织加热，达到杀灭癌细胞的温度，以治疗恶性肿瘤。

N：RFA is a treatment method that introduces the heat into the tumor to kill the tumor cells.

患者：那要达到多少度？

P：How high will the temperature go?

护士：肝脏肿瘤射频的靶温度设置一般为 80～105 ℃，人体最适合的温度为 37 ℃左右，当处于 41～43 ℃时，正常组织能耐受此温度不受损伤，达 60 ℃时细胞会很快死亡。

N：In the targeted tumor area, the temperature of the RFA is usually set at 80 ℃ to 105 ℃. The most suitable temperature for normal tissues is about 37 ℃. Normal tissues can withstand the heat ranging from 41 ℃ to 43 ℃. If the temperature reaches 60 ℃, the cells will die soon.

患者：那对正常的组织有损伤吗？

P：Is there any damage to normal tissues?

护士：为了确保肿瘤完全消融，消融范围要超过肿瘤边缘 5 mm 以上，一般来说不会造成周围器官的损伤。

N：In order to get complete necrosis of tumor, the ablation area is required to cover at least 5 mm more than the outer edge of the tumor. In general, it will not hurt the surrounding organs.

患者：治疗过程中痛吗？

P：Is there any pain during the treatment?

护士：治疗过程中会给您使用止痛药的，不会有太疼痛的感受。

N：You may experience some pain or discomfort, but the doctor will give you some painkiller to help you.

患者：好的，谢谢。

P：OK. Thank you.

护士：治疗过程中可能会感觉比较热。

N：You may feel hot during the treatment.

患者：会很热吗？

P：Will it be very hot?

护士：会比您的体温要高，您会出汗。

N：It will be higher than your body temperature. You may sweat.

患者：好的。

P：OK.

护士：治疗要在 B 超或 CT 下进行，您需要提前 4 小时禁食。

N：We use ultrasound or CT to guide the surgery. You should fast for 4 hours before the surgery.

患者：好的。

P：OK.

护士：您的治疗在下午两点，我们会提前通知卫勤人员送您去治疗室。

N：Your surgery will start at 2 p. m. , we will inform the medical staff in advance to escort you to the therapeutic room.

患者：好的。谢谢！

P：OK. Thank you.

护士：我们应该做的。

N：It's my pleasure.

[**Phrases**]

a brief introduction	简要介绍
range from . . . to	范围是……
therapeutic room	治疗室
in advance	提前

5. Health Education for Patients Before Argon-Helium Cryoablation

氩氦冷冻消融术前患者的健康教育

[Glossary]

argon-helium cryoablation	氩氦冷冻消融术
argon-helium knife	氩氦刀
chemotherapy	化疗
cryotherapy	冷冻治疗
radiotherapy	放疗
minimally invasive	微创
anaesthetic	麻醉药
hyperthermia	热疗
hemostatic medicine	止血药物

[Scenario]

患者：李护士，我是今天刚入院的患者，医生要给我做冷冻治疗，我想了解一下。

P：Nurse Li, I am a new patient and was scheduled to have a cryotherapy today. Could you please tell me more details about this treatment?

护士：好的，氩氦冷冻消融术是一种微创超低温冷冻消融肿瘤的先进技术，也叫作"氩氦刀"。它在 CT 或 B 超定位引导下将氩氦刀准确穿刺进入肿瘤内，先用氩气，刀尖会急速膨胀产生制冷作用，在 15 秒内将病变组织冷冻至零下 140 ℃～零下 170 ℃，持续15～20 分钟后，关闭氩气，再使用氦气，氦气在刀尖急速膨胀，急速加热处于超低温状态的病变组织，使其温度从零下 140 ℃上升至零上 20～40 ℃，从而施行快速热疗。持续 3～5 分钟之后，再重复一次，可

杀死病变组织。其降温及升温的速度、时间，摧毁区
域的尺寸与形状等，由 B 超或 CT 等实时监测，计算
机精确设定和控制。

N：Well, argon-helium cryoablation is an advanced
minimally invasive therapy that ablates tumors with
ultra-low temperature. This treatment method is also
called "argon-helium knife". The argon-helium knife
punctures accurately into the tumor under the
guidance of CT or ultrasound. Argon is first rapidly
expanded on the tip of the knife to generate a cooling
effect, which can freeze the lesion tissues to minus
140 ℃～minus 170 ℃ in 15 seconds. After 15 to 20
minutes, argon is turned off and helium is released on
the tip of the knife to generate a rapid heating effect
to the lesion tissues to rapidly elevate the temperature
from minus 140 ℃ to 20 ～ 40 ℃, for rapid
hyperthermia. After 3 to 5 minutes, repeat the
procedure to kill the lesion tissues. The rate and time
of temperature changes, size and shape of the desired
target tissues are all monitored by ultrasound or CT in
real-time mode, and they are set and controlled
precisely by the computer.

患者：这样的温度我受不了吧！
P：I don't think I can tolerate such a temperature change!

护士：不用担心，只是肿瘤部位温度有变化，您不会有太多
感觉。
N：Oh, don't worry about it too much. The temperature
change only occurs in the targeted area, you can
hardly feel it.

患者：那就好。
P：That's good.

护士：它对其他部位组织无损伤或损伤极小，这是有别于

放疗和化疗的独特优点。

N：This treatment has no or minimal damage to other tissues，which is the unique advantage compared with radiotherapy and chemotherapy.

患者：谢谢，那我要注意一些什么吗？

P：Thank you，what should I pay attention to？

护士：治疗前需要禁食 4 小时，术前医生常规会给你开点止血药，现在请在病房等待。

N：You should not eat or drink 4 hours before the treatment. The doctor usually gives you some hemostatic medicine before the surgery. Now please wait in the ward.

患者：谢谢，我现在没有那么紧张了。

P：Thank you. I am much relieved now.

护士：不客气。

N：You are welcome.

[Phrases]

control precisely	精确控制
turn off	关闭
under the guidance of	在……的引导下

6. Health Education for Patients Before Microwave Ablation
微波消融术前患者的健康教育

[Glossary]

microwave ablation	微波消融
mechanism	机理
skin puncture	皮肤穿刺
microwave oven	微波炉
surrounding tissue	周围组织
thermal effect	热效应
hemostatic	止血药

[Scenario]

患者：孙护士，医生确定我的手术方案是微波消融术。

P：Nurse Sun，my doctor confirmed that the treatment method is microwave ablation.

护士：那太好了。

N：That is great.

患者：微波消融术是不是和微波炉原理一样的？

P：How does microwave ablation work? Does it use the same mechanism as microwave oven?

护士：让我为你讲解一下。

N：Let me explain it.

患者：那太感谢了。

P：Thank you.

护士：微波消融术是利用专用治疗针，在超声或 CT 引导下，经皮肤穿刺直接进入肿瘤病灶，利用微波炉一样的热效应原理，使肿瘤组织局部在几分钟内达到 60～100 ℃ 的高温，达到"烧死"肿瘤细胞的目的，而

　　周围组织损伤较少,因为单针消融范围的直径只有
　　3 cm 左右。

N：Microwave ablation method uses a special needle to puncture through the skin into the tumor under the guidance of ultrasound or CT. The mechanism is just like the thermal effect of microwave oven. The temperature of the targeted tumor tissue area is elevated to 60～100 ℃ within a few minutes. The very high temperature in tumor area can "burn" tumor cells to death,but the damage to surrounding normal tissues is limited as the diameter of the ablation area of single needle is about 3 cm.

患者：谢谢,那我要注意什么吗?

P：Thank you. What should I pay attention to?

护士：治疗前需要禁食 4 小时,术前医生会给你开点常规
　　　止血药,现在请在病房等待,医生会在你签手术知情
　　　同意书时为你详细讲解的。

N：You should not eat anything for 4 hours before the surgery. The doctor will give you some routine hemostatic medicine. Now you just need to stay in the ward. The doctor will explain to you the details when you sign the informed consent.

患者：谢谢!

P：Thank you so much.

护士：不客气!

N：You are welcome.

[Phrases]

pay attention to　　　　　　　　注意

tumor tissue　　　　　　　　　　肿瘤组织

7. Health Education for Patients Treated by Percutaneous Ethanol Injection
经皮肝穿刺无水乙醇瘤内注射
治疗患者的健康教育

[Glossary]

absolute ethanol	无水乙醇
percutaneous	经皮的
dizziness	眩晕

[Scenario]

护士：3床王阿姨，医生有没有跟您说明天酒精治疗？

N：Ms. Wang, has your doctor told you about your percutaneous ethanol injection treatment tomorrow?

患者：说了。

P：Yes, he has.

护士：好的，我现在给您做术前宣教，请您仔细听好，有疑问可以随时打断我。

N：OK, I will give you the preoperative education. Please listen carefully and interrupt me whenever you have any questions.

患者：我知道了。

P：OK, I will.

护士：这个治疗方法是采用经皮肝穿刺，在其尖端达肝内病灶后注射无水乙醇，使病变组织发生凝固性坏死。

N：The doctor performs this procedure by puncturing a special needle through your skin into the liver tumor. Once the needle is in the tumor, the doctor will inject absolute ethanol into it to kill the tumor cells.

患者：无水乙醇？ 不是酒精吗？

P：Absolute ethanol? Not alcohol?

护士：无水乙醇就是酒精，它是纯度为99%的酒精。

N：Absolute ethanol is alcohol，with the purity of 99%.

患者：打这么高浓度的酒精，一定会不舒服的吧？

P：Will I feel uncomfortable when such high concentration of alcohol is injected into my body?

护士：王阿姨，不要担心，之前医生通过检查已经了解您的身体状况，在身体条件允许的情况下才会给您治疗。一般治疗下来，大多数患者情况都不错，只有小部分患者会出现上腹部不适、疼痛、呕吐、头晕等症状，我们会对症处理的。

N：Ms. Wang，don't worry. The doctor has evaluated your physical condition and make sure you will tolerate this procedure. Most patients can tolerate this procedure well. However，some patients may experience some degree of abdominal discomfort，pain，vomiting，dizziness and other symptoms. The doctor will treat those symptoms accordingly.

患者：好的。

P：That's good.

护士：如果您有什么不懂的地方，可以随时问我。

N：Don't hesitate to ask me if you have any questions.

患者：谢谢，我大概了解了。

P：Thank you，I think I have a general idea of it now.

[Phrases]

abdominal discomfort	腹部不适
concentration of alcohol	酒精浓度
preoperative education	术前宣教
interrupt sb.	打断某人

8. Health Education for Patients with Liver Abscess Treated by Drainage Under Ultrasound Guidance
超声引导下肝脓肿置管引流患者的健康教育

[Glossary]

liver abscess	肝脓肿
bacterial	细菌性的
chill	寒战
percutaneous	经皮的
cavity	腔;洞
blood vessel	血管

[Scenario]

患者：李护士,我今天发热了,体温又是 38 ℃,我怎么老是发热?

P：Nurse Li, I have a fever today and my temperature is 38 ℃. Why do I always have a fever?

护士：刘叔叔,这是您的疾病引起的,您的肝脏受感染后,因未及时处理而形成脓肿。有细菌性和阿米巴性两种,您是细菌引起的。临床上一般都会出现寒战、高热、肝区疼痛、肝肿大。

N：Mr. Liu, your fever is caused by infection in your liver. The liver formed an abscess as the infection hadn't been treated promptly. Bacteria and ameba are common microorganisms that cause liver abscess. You are most likely to have a bacterial liver abscess. The common symptoms of liver abscess include chill, fever, liver pain and liver enlargement.

患者：那我的病能治好吗? 这样下去,会不会有生命危险?

P：Is it serious? Will I recover?

护士：处理及时是会治疗好的。

N：The liver abscess can be cured if it is treated appropriately.

患者：现在有什么好办法呢？

P：How to treat?

护士：在超声引导下肝脓肿穿刺引流这个治疗方法在临床上已经非常成熟了，已发展成为治疗肝脓肿的首选。

N：The liver abscess is commonly treated by ultrasound guided drainage. It is a mature procedure in clinic and has been the first choice of treatment.

患者：这个是手术治疗吗？

P：Is this a surgery?

护士：不是，这是一个微创治疗，它经皮肝穿刺置管引流，用于脓肿直径 5～10 cm 者，用 PTCD 引流管置入脓腔，引流管接负压，必要时每天抽吸并冲洗。它的创伤性小、定位准确、危险性系数低，在 B 超引导下可以避开血管、胆管及重要脏器，达到安全治疗的目的。

N：Not really. This is a minimally invasive procedure. We call it percutaneous transhepatic catheter drainage or PTCD. This procedure is usually used for the abscess of 5 to 10 cm in size. In this procedure a drainage tube is inserted into the abscess cavity. The drainage tube is connected to negative pressure to suck and wash out the abscess content. We can repeat this procedure every day if necessary. This procedure has a minimally invasive incision；it accurately targets the lesion without touching blood vessels，the bile duct and important organs by using ultrasound. All in all，this treatment method is very safe.

患者：效果如何？

P：How effective is this treatment?

护士：疗效可靠，并发症发生率低。

N：In general, this is an effective and safe treatment method with very few complications.

患者：我要一直带着引流管吗?

P：Do I have to carry the drainage tube all the time?

护士：不用，等脓腔变小，感染控制住了，医生会根据您的恢复情况进行拔管。

N：No. Once the abscess is controlled, meaning the size becomes smaller, the doctor will pull out the drainage tube according to your condition.

患者：那我还要注意什么?

P：What else should I pay attention to?

护士：您需要加强营养，多吃多种维生素，以改善肝功能。

N：You need to improve your liver function by eating nutritious foods and vitamins.

患者：谢谢。

P：OK. Thank you.

[Phrases]

be caused by	由……引起
be cured	被治愈
first choice	首选
insert into	置入
negative pressure	负压

9. Health Education for Patients in Perioperative Period of Vertebroplasty
椎体成形术围手术期患者的健康教育

[Glossary]

vertebroplasty	椎体成形术
bone cement	骨水泥
medical material	医用材料
solidification	凝固
vertebral body	椎体
hypoxemia	低血氧
hypotension	低血压
arrhythmia	心律失常
pulmonary hypertension	肺动脉高压
coagulation function	凝血功能
incidence	发生率

[Scenario]

患者：张护士，今天主任查房，说要给我打骨水泥。我想咨询一下这是什么？

P：Nurse Zhang, my doctor told me that he will do a procedure called bone cement. I would like to know more about this.

护士：高伯伯，骨水泥是一种用于骨头的医用材料，由于它的部分物理性质以及凝固后的外观和性状颇像建筑、装修用的白水泥，便有了如此的名称。

N：Mr. Gao, the bone cement is a special medical material used for some bone diseases. The name derives from part of its physical properties and the appearance and character after solidification that are similar to the white cement used for construction and decoration.

患者：我知道了。

P：Oh, I see.

护士：它主要用来解除或减轻您的疼痛、加固椎体和防止椎体进一步压缩塌陷。

N：It is mainly used to relieve your pain, strengthen the vertebral body and prevent the collapse of the vertebral body.

患者：那太好了，长期的疼痛让我总是失眠。

P：That's great. It will solve my insomnia caused by long-lasting pain.

护士：等治疗结束，您的疼痛在一定程度上会得到缓解。

N：Your pain will be relieved to some extent when the treatment is done.

患者：这个治疗医生会怎么做，你能给我说说吗？

P：Could you explain this procedure to me in detail?

护士：它是用骨穿刺针在透视监视下行椎体穿刺后，将骨水泥注入病变椎体内，从而达到治疗的目的。

N：In this procedure, a needle is punctured into the lesion area of vertebral body under X-ray, then the bone cement is injected into the lesion.

患者：有什么副作用吗？

P：Any side effects?

护士：有可能会有骨水泥植入综合征，目前对 BCIS 的定义尚未明确界定，其临床表现包括低血氧、低血压、心律失常、肺动脉高压、凝血功能改变等。

N：It may cause bone cement implantation syndrome (BCIS). To date, the definition of BCIS has not been clearly made. The clinical manifestations include hypoxemia, hypotension, arrhythmia, pulmonary hypertension, changes in coagulation function and so on.

患者：哦！

P：Oh!

护士：您不要太担心，发生率并不高。

N：Please do not worry too much. The incidence of BCIS is not that high in our practice.

患者：我相信医生，我还需要做什么？

P：I have confidence in doctors，what else do I need to do?

护士：骨水泥手术后可以吃易于消化且富含营养素的食物。之后可以进食高蛋白、高脂肪、高碳水化合物，并富含维生素和矿物质的食物，有利于骨的修复和愈合。术后组织的修复和生长将消耗较多的钙、镁、锌等矿物，应注意从食物中补充。

N：In general，you should eat digestible foods with rich nutrients just after the surgery，then eat foods that are rich in protein，fat，carbohydrate，vitamins and minerals in order to help vertebral tissue repair after the surgery. The repair and growth of the vertebral tissue requires a lot of calcium，magnesium，zinc and other minerals.

患者：好的，我都记住了。谢谢。

P：OK，I see. Thank you.

护士：没事，如果您忘记了可以再问我。

N：You are welcome. Please feel free to ask me if you have any questions.

[Phrases]

physical property	物理性质
be similar to	类似于
relieve pain	减轻疼痛

10. Health Education for Patients Undergoing Transjugular Intrahepatic Portosystemic Stent Shunt

经颈静脉穿刺肝内门-体静脉支撑架
分流手术患者的健康教育

[Glossary]

transjugular	经颈静脉
intrahepatic	肝内的
portosystemic	门体静脉
bloated	胀的
ascites	腹水
cirrhosis	肝硬化
diuretic	利尿剂;利尿的

[Scenario]

患者：护士，为什么我用了那么多药物，肚子还是那么胀？我现在非常难受，什么都吃不下去了，我感觉躺下去就不舒服。

P：Nurse，why is my stomach still so bloated even after I have been taking so many medications? I'm too uncomfortable to eat anything, especially when I lie down.

护士：李先生，我知道您非常难受，我建议您选择半卧位，这样也许会舒服点。您的肚子里面有大量的腹水，而腹水的产生是因为腹腔内游离液体的过量积聚，这是由于您肝硬化太严重了，腹水比较顽固，所以药物控制的效果，您觉得不明显。

N：Mr. Li, I understand your condition. Would you like to try a semi-recumbent position? This position may make you feel better. The reason you have such a bloated stomach is that a large amount of ascites accumulates due to your serious liver cirrhosis. As a result，you could barely feel the effect of the medication.

患者：原来是这样，那就没有什么办法给我解决了吗？

P：Oh，I see. Are there any methods to relieve my condition?

护士：会有解决的办法，比如经颈静脉穿刺肝内门-体静脉支撑架分流术(TIPPS)。

N：Of course，we use a method called TIPPS to help our patients with your condition.

患者：这是什么治疗？

P：What's this treatment?

护士：经颈静脉穿刺肝内门-体静脉支撑架分流术。

N：TIPPS stands for transjugular intrahepatic portosystemic stent-shunt.

患者：我没有听过，你能给我讲讲吗？

P：This is something new to me. Could you explain this method to me please?

护士：腹水是由门脉高压所致，TIPPS 利用分流原理，通过一系列介入器具的使用，在肝实质内肝静脉与门静脉间建立起人工分流通道，从而降低门脉压力、减少或消除腹水症状。

N：The ascites is caused by portal hypertension. In TIPPS method，a series of interventional device is used to divert blood from portal vein to hepatic vein to reduce the portal pressure. That will help you control or even get rid of the ascites.

患者：这样就能解决我的腹胀了吗？

P：Will it cure my bloating?

护士：如果治疗很成功，应该能缓解您现在的症状。

N：If the treatment is successful，it should be able to alleviate your current symptoms.

患者：谢谢，这让我感觉好受多了，希望医生尽快给我
　　　治疗。

P：Thank you. It makes me feel much better. I hope the
　　doctor can give me the treatment as soon as possible.

护士：等您做完所有的检查，应该就会安排治疗的，这期间
　　　医生会给您些利尿剂，来缓解您腹胀的情况。

N：The doctor will schedule your treatment as soon as your
　　pre-operation examination is completed. During your
　　waiting period, the doctor will prescribe some diuretic
　　medicines to relieve your bloating.

患者：是的，我一直都在吃。

P：Yes, I've been taking that medicine.

护士：好的，如果您还有什么疑问，可以随时问我，我叫
　　　春雨。

N：OK. If you have further questions, please feel free to
　　ask me. My name is Chunyu.

[Phrases]

lie down	躺下
semi-recumbent position	半卧位
a large amount of	大量的
accumulation	积累
a series of	一系列的
portal vein	门静脉
interventional device	介入装置
shunt	分流渠道
hepatic vein	肝静脉

11. Health Education for Patients Implanted with Radioactive Particles
放射性粒子植入患者的健康教育

[Glossary]

seeds implantation	粒子植入治疗
implant	植入
radioactive	放射性的
particle	粒子
tumor cell	肿瘤细胞
penetration	穿透
proliferate	增殖

[Scenario]

护士：您好！我是您的责任护士王芳。

N：Hello! I'm your primary nurse. My name is Wang Fang.

患者：你好！

P：Hello!

护士：您今天需要做粒子植入治疗，医生已经开出医嘱。

N：According to the doctor's medical orders, you need to receive I‑125 seeds implantation today.

患者：好的。

P：OK.

护士：请问您之前进行过粒子植入治疗吗？

N：Have you ever received the seeds implantation before?

患者：没有。

P：Not yet.

护士：那我现在给您讲解一下。

N：Now I will tell you some details about it.

患者：好的。

P：Good.

护士：粒子植入治疗是在超声或 CT 引导下将一定数量的粒子植入瘤体，植入瘤体内的放射性粒子能连续不断地发出射线，持续照射破坏肿瘤细胞核的 DNA，使肿瘤细胞失去增殖能力。

N：The seeds implantation is a treatment method by implanting a certain number of radioactive particles in the tumor under the guidance of ultrasound or CT. The radioactive particles implanted in the tumor can continuously emit radiation and damage the DNA of tumor cells. Thus, the tumor cells lose their ability to proliferate.

患者：粒子有射线，那我还能和家人住一起吗？

P：Can I still live with my family once the radioactive particles are implanted in my body?

护士：射线的穿透距离非常有限，您还是可以和家人住一起的，不过建议不要和婴幼儿以及孕妇过多接触。

N：That would not be a problem since the penetration of the radiation is very limited. It will not harm the people living with you. But you should avoid touching infants or pregnant women frequently.

患者：治疗过程中痛吗？

P：Is it painful during the treatment?

护士：大部分患者没有疼痛的感觉，医生也会根据治疗中的情况以及您的主诉合理使用止痛药。

N：Most patients won't feel the pain, and the doctor will give you painkillers in the treatment according to your situation.

患者：好的，谢谢。

P：OK. Thank you.

护士：治疗要在 B 超或 CT 下进行，您需要提前 4 小时禁食。

N：The procedure will be performed under the guidance of ultrasound or CT and you should fast for 4 hours prior to the treatment.

患者：好的。

P：No problem.

护士：您的治疗下午两点开始，我们会提前通知卫勤人员送您去治疗室。

N：Your treatment will start at 2 p.m. and we will inform the medical staff in advance to take you to the therapeutic room.

患者：好的。谢谢！

P：OK，thank you.

护士：我们应该做的。

N：My pleasure!

[Phrases]

in advance	提前
medical order	医嘱

12. Health Education for Patients After Intravenous Infusion Catheter Implantation
静脉输液管植入术后患者的健康教育

[Glossary]

wound	伤口
bleeding	出血
painkiller	止疼药
incision	切口
maintenance	维护
swelling	肿胀

[Scenario]

护士：阿姨，您回来了，感觉怎么样啊？让我看一下您的伤口。阿姨，伤口挺好的，没有出血。回来先卧床休息为主，不可以剧烈活动，有什么不舒服就按铃呼叫我们，我们也会经常过来看您的。

N：How are you doing? Please let me take a look at your wound. The wound is in good condition with no bleeding. Rest properly and avoid strenuous activities. We will check on you periodically. Please bell us if you need help.

患者：但是我现在感觉伤口有点酸痛。

P：But I feel a little pain in the wound.

护士：阿姨，手术过后由于输液港植入初期的局部刺激，您可能感觉伤口酸痛不适，一般 1～2 天可自行缓解。您可以听听音乐，看看报纸或者手机视频，多跟家人聊聊天，这样有利于转移注意力，减轻疼痛感。如果您实在忍受不了疼痛，那就及时按铃，我们会将您的情况告诉医生，医生会给您使用止疼药的。

N：You may feel some pain and discomfort in the wound area because of the irritation of the implanted infusion port. It may last for several days, but it will go away eventually. You can divert your attention by listening to the music, reading newspapers or watching videos on your cell phone or chat with your family members. If those do not help and you still feel the pain, please tell us in time and the doctor will give you some painkillers.

患者：那这个术后要注意什么呢？

P：What should I pay attention to after the surgery?

护士：您最近需要保证舒适、良好的睡眠。这个过程中您只能擦浴，待局部拆线伤口愈合后才可以淋浴。在切口完全愈合前，穿刺侧上肢尽量内收，减少剧烈活动，避免植入处上肢做剧烈外展动作及打篮球、引体向上、托举哑铃等持重锻炼，避免负重，并保持切口及其周围干燥，以降低切口裂开及感染的风险。这个输液港一般 10～14 天拆线，对生活影响不大。您出院回家后，每个月要到正规医院进行一次冲管和维护，每次都要抽出回血，保证导管是通的。伤口愈合后就能恢复正常生活。如果出现红、肿、热、痛，及时去医院就诊。

N：Presently, you need to ensure good sleeps. During this period, you can only have sponge baths, and shower is not allowed until local wound is healed. Before the incision is completely healed, try to keep the involved upper arm close to your body as much as possible. Do not take strenuous exercises or stretch the upper limb. You should avoid activities such as playing basketball, doing pull-ups, lifting dumbbells or weight-bearing exercises. You should keep the incision wound area dry to reduce the risk of wound dehiscence or infection. It will be 10 to 14 days before we take out the stitches. The infusion port usually do not cause troubles in your daily life. After you are discharged，you need to come back to the hospital once a month for the port maintenance such as tube flush and withdraw some blood from the tube to ensure that the catheter is not obstructed. Your daily life can go back to normal once the wound is healed. Please come back to see your doctor immediately if you have a fever or pain，or see redness or swelling in wound area.

患者：好的，谢谢护士。

P：OK，thanks.

护士：那您好好休息。

N：You're welcome. Have a good rest.

[Phrases]

infusion port	输液港
divert attention	转移注意力
ensure a good sleep	保证良好睡眠
sponge bath	擦浴
go back to normal	恢复正常

13. Health Education for Patients of Drug-Loaded Microspheres with Tumor Interventional Therapy
肿瘤介入治疗中载药微球患者的健康教育

[Glossary]

microparticle	微球;微粒
formulation	制剂
starch	淀粉
chitosan	壳聚糖
carrier	载体
doxorubicin	多柔比星(阿霉素)
epirubicin	表柔比星(表阿霉素)
irinotecan	伊立替康
embolization	栓塞
toxicity	毒性
enzyme	酶

[Scenario]

护士：夏先生，您好，我是您的责任护士丽丽。您需要进行介入治疗，我来跟您说一下注意事项。

N: Hello, Mr. Xia. I'm your primary nurse, Li Li. You are scheduled for an interventional treatment. Let me tell you some details about it.

患者：好的，丽丽，我还准备去找你了解一下呢，我明天有一个新药，以前都没听说过。

P: OK, Li Li. I am just going to come to you. I will receive a new drug tomorrow, but I haven't heard of it before.

护士：您说的是载药微球吧，您有什么不懂的，我来解释给您听。

N：Are you talking about the drug-loaded microsphere? What do you want to know about? I'll explain it to you.

患者：我想知道载药微球的作用原理，以及用的什么药。

P：I would like to know how this drug-loaded microsphere works, and which drug is loaded.

护士：好。药物微球是一种新型药物制剂，它是利用淀粉、壳聚糖、聚乳酸、明胶等高分子聚合物材料作为载体，将固体或液体药物包裹而形成的微小的球状实体的固体骨架物，其直径大小不一，一般在 100～300 μm，甚至更大，属于基质型骨架微粒。

N：All right. Drug-loaded microsphere is a new type of drug formulation which uses starch, chitosan, polylactic acid, gelatin and other polymer materials as carrier. It encapsulates solid or liquid drugs in a tiny globular entity. Its diameter is generally 100～300 μm, sometimes larger. It's a kind of matrix scaffold microsphere.

患者：听起来很复杂，那可以用哪些药呢？

P：Sounds complicated. Specifically, what drugs can be used by this drug-loaded microsphere?

护士：载药微球可以负载多柔比星、表柔比星、伊立替康等多种化疗药物，在肝癌等恶性肿瘤中，起到栓塞与局部高浓度化疗的联合作用，使患者全身毒副作用大大降低，同时也可以显著提高进展期肝癌的客观有效率和疾病控制率。

N：It can carry doxorubicin, epirubicin, irinotecan and other chemotherapeutic agents. In the treatment of liver cancers and other malignant tumors, it combines embolization with chemotherapy with high local concentration, which greatly reduces toxicity and meanwhile, significantly improves the efficacy and disease control rate of liver cancers in progressive stage.

患者：那它的副作用大吗?

P: How about the side effects?

护士：载药微球作为一种新型给药技术,既能通过调节和控制药物的释放速度实现长效的目的,又能保护药物不受体内酶的影响而降解,掩盖药物的不良口味,减少给药次数和药物刺激,降低毒性和不良反应,提高疗效。此外,微球还与某些细胞组织有特殊亲和性,能被器官组织的网状内皮系统所内吞或被细胞融合,集中于靶区逐步扩散释出药物或被溶酶体中的酶降解而释出药物,从而起到靶向治疗的作用。

N: As a new drug delivery technique, the drug-loaded microsphere can improve efficacy by regulating and controlling release speed of drugs, and prevent drugs from degrading by enzyme. It can also avoid the unpleasant taste of the drug itself, decrease the frequency of administration, reduce drug stimulation, toxicity and other side effects, and thus improve the drug efficacy. In addition, the drug-loaded microsphere has special affinity with specific cells and tissues by means of being engulfed by reticuloendothelial system or fused by cells. The drug is then concentrated at the target area and gradually dispersed or released by enzymatic degradation of the lysosome, in this way it plays the role of targeted therapy.

患者：你讲得很详细也很清楚,我明白了,谢谢你的解释。

P: I see. Thank you for your detailed explanation.

护士：不用谢,这是我应该做的。祝您明天手术成功。

N: You are welcome, this is my duty. Wish you a successful operation tomorrow.

[**Phrases**]

interventional treatment	介入治疗
drug-loaded microparticle	载药微球
polylactic acid	聚乳酸
polymer material	聚合物材料
globular entity	球状实体
matrix scaffold microparticle	基质型骨架微粒
high concentration	高浓度
drug delivery technique	给药技术
drug stimulation	药物刺激
drug toxicity	药物毒性
enzymatic degradation	酶降解

14. Health Education for Patients After Interventional Therapy with Indwelling Catheter
介入术后留鞘泵疗患者的健康教育

[Glossary]

embolization	栓塞
indwell	植入
arterial	动脉的
pump	泵入
postoperatively	术后
prolong	延长
injection	注射
hematoma	血肿
nausea	恶心
antiemetic	止吐药
extravasation	外渗
extubation	拔管

[Scenario]

护士：王芳，今天要做介入治疗对吗？

N：Wang Fang, you are scheduled for an intervention treatment today, right?

患者：是的，听说这次要留根管子，要做什么用啊？

P：Yes, I heard that a tube is going to be left in my body this time. What's it for?

护士：对的，会留一根管子，回来会继续泵药的。因为单纯的栓塞对您的基本效果并不明显，需要加大剂量。术后留置动脉导管泵注化疗药，可使单次注射时间延长，增加肿瘤局部药物浓度并延长作用时间，从而达到更好的治疗效果。

N：Yes. A tube will be left in your body after the surgery in order to pump chemotherapeutic drugs continuously. We need to increase the drug dosage because the simple embolization treatment was not effective for you. Pumping chemotherapeutic drugs through the indwelling arterial catheter postoperatively can achieve a better treatment outcome by prolonging single injection time，increasing local drug concentration and extending the time of drug efficacy.

患者：那有什么要注意的吗？

P：What shall I pay attention to?

护士：因为需要输注化疗药物，化疗药物一般都会引起胃肠反应，如恶心、呕吐，如果反应比较大，我们会根据情况给您用一些止吐药。

N：Because chemotherapeutic drugs will be infused，generally they will cause gastrointestinal reactions，such as nausea and vomiting. If the reaction is serious，we will give you some antiemetics depending on the situation.

患者：这个管子主要作用就是化疗吗？

P：Is this tube mainly used for chemotherapy?

护士：是的。

N：Yes.

患者：那我需要注意什么吗？身上留着一根管子让我很害怕。

P：Anything else I need to pay attention to? I am scared to keep a tube in my body.

护士：阿姨，您不要太害怕。这根管子并不是很粗，而且为了您的治疗，这个是非常必要的。用药期间您要注意导管有无扭曲、受压、堵管和外渗，穿刺口不要接触水，要保持干燥清洁，以防止感染，我们也会每天按时查看。另外，您有任何不舒服都可以随时告诉护士,护士 24 小时值班。

N：Don't worry too much. This tube is thin, and it is necessary for your treatment. During the medication, you should inspect the catheter for kink, compression, blockage and extravasation, keep the wound dry and clean to prevent possible infection. Also, we will check it regularly every day. In addition, if you have any discomfort, just tell us, we are on 24-hour duty.

患者：那我这个管子什么时候能拔掉呢？

P：When will this tube be pulled out?

护士：这个药用完之后医生就会过来拔管的,拔管后要用沙袋压迫 2 小时以预防出血。拔管后要注意观察局部有无出血和血肿,如果有出血,我们会给您重新加压包扎,血肿 24 小时后可进行热敷,以促进吸收。

N：The doctor will pull the catheter out once your drug infusion is completed. You should press the wound for 2 hours with a sandbag to prevent bleeding after extubation. Then we will examine if local bleeding or hematoma occurs. If bleeding happens, we will wrap the wound up again with pressure. In case of hematoma, warm compress can be used after 24 hours to promote absorption.

患者：好的,我明白了,谢谢你。

P：All right, I see. Thank you.

护士：不用谢。

N：You are welcome.

[Phrases]

interventional operation	介入手术
increase the dosage	增加剂量
drug concentration	药物浓度
treatment outcome	治疗效果

gastrointestinal reaction	胃肠道反应
prevent infection	防止感染
warm compress	热敷
promote absorption	促进吸收

15. Health Education for Patients After Endoscopic Retrograde Cholangiopancreatography
经内镜逆行胰胆管造影术后患者的健康教育

[Glossary]

bile	胆汁
amylase	淀粉酶
infect	感染
duodenum	十二指肠
lung	肺
uterus	子宫
pancreatitis	胰腺炎

[Scenario]

护士：张阿姨，您现在感觉好点了吗？

N：Ms. Zhang, do you feel better now?

患者：不，我感觉鼻子痒痒的，很难受。

P：No, my nose is itchy, I feel very uncomfortable.

护士：您刚刚做完 ERCP 术，会有一些不适感，这个非常正常。

N：You have just finished ERCP. There will be some discomfort, which is normal.

患者：这个管子什么时候能拔掉啊？

P：When can this catheter be pulled out?

护士：现在暂时不能拔掉，因为留置鼻胆管主要是为了引流出感染的胆汁并消除胆胰反流，有效控制炎症。留置管道期间，暂时不能吃任何食物，等血淀粉酶的结果出来才能确定是否能吃东西。

N：This nasal catheter should not be pulled out at this moment because we use it to drain the infected bile and to prevent pancreatobiliary reflux in order to control the inflammation. During this time you should not eat any food until your blood amylase level returns to normal.

患者：血淀粉酶是什么？

P：What is blood amylase?

护士：血淀粉酶是一种主要由胰腺分泌的消化酶，另外，十二指肠、肺、子宫、泌乳期的乳腺等器官也有少量分泌。血清淀粉酶活性测定主要用于急性胰腺炎的诊断。

N：Blood amylase is a digestive enzyme which is mainly secreted by the pancreas. Additionally, a small amount of blood amylase comes from the duodenum, lung, uterus, mammary gland of breastfeeding women and other organs as well. The activity of serum amylase is mainly used for the diagnosis of acute pancreatitis.

患者：什么时候可以抽血？

P：When is the blood test performed?

护士：术后您需要卧床休息，禁食 24 小时。术后 3 小时及次日凌晨分别查血淀粉酶，若淀粉酶正常，无腹痛、发热、黄疸等情况方可进食。由清流质过渡到低脂流质，再到低脂半流质，避免摄入粗纤维食物，防止对术后十二指肠乳头的摩擦导致渗血，一周后可进食普食，但如果严重的话，需适当延长禁食和卧床时间，建立静脉输液通路，给予支持治疗。

N：You must fast for 24 hours and stay in bed for several hours after the surgery. Your blood amylase will be analyzed 3 hours and the next morning after the surgery. You can eat foods if the amylase is normal, and no abdominal pain, fever or jaundice presents. You should gradually convert from a clear-fluid diet to a low-fat liquid diet, and then to a low-fat semi-liquid diet, and avoid intake of crude fiber to reduce the friction to the duodenal papilla, which may cause bleeding. A week later, you may have a normal diet. However, if your condition is serious, you ought to extend time of fasting and bed resting, and establish the intravenous infusion pathway as a supportive treatment.

患者：那我还需要注意什么? 我希望能尽快拔管。

P：What else should I pay attention to? I wish the catheter would be removed as soon as possible.

护士：我们需要固定鼻胆管。活动及睡觉时，保护好导管，以防意外脱出。如怀疑导管有少许脱出，不宜强行往里送导管，及时告诉我就可以了。我们会随时观察胆汁引流情况，确保充分引流，每日我也会观察并记录引流液的量、颜色、性质。一般每日引流量在 $200\sim800$ ml，如若引流量减少或无胆汁引出，可能是因为导管堵塞或脱出，但您不用担心，我们会对症处理的，不会危及您的生命。

N：We need to keep the catheter in the right position all the time. Please take good care of the catheter during daytime activity and sleep to prevent it from accidentally sliding out. If you suspect the catheter is sliding out, please let us know and do not attempt to put the catheter back by yourself. We will observe constantly the outflow of the bile to ensure adequate drainage. Besides, we will observe and record the volume, color and nature of the drainage fluid every day. Generally, the volume of daily drainage is around 200 to 800 ml. If the volume is markedly reduced or no drainage is observed, then catheter blockage or sliding may have occurred. In that case，we will deal with it timely. Don't worry，it will not threaten your life.

患者：太感谢了!
P：Thanks a lot!
护士：不客气。
N：You're welcome.

[Phrases]

intravenous infusion	静脉输液
supportive treatment	支持治疗

16. Doctor and Patient's Dialogue in the Operating Room
手术室医患情景对话

手术前

Before the operation

[Glossary]

DSA room	导管室
intervention ward	介入病房
hepatic arterial	肝动脉的
chemoembolization	化疗栓塞
femoral artery	股动脉
angiography	血管造影术
lesion	病灶
anesthesia	麻醉

[Scenario]

护士：您好，我们这里是导管室或者叫介入手术室。我是今天的当班护士，我姓宋。请问您叫什么名字？住在哪个病区？几楼几床？

N：Hello，this is the conduit room or interventional operating room. I am the nurse on duty today，my last name is Song. May I have your name? And which ward are you from?

患者：我叫张建，住在介入病房，21 号楼 3 楼 3 床。

P：My name is Zhang Jian，I stay in the intervention ward，building 21，3rd floor，bed 3.

（护士核查患者的基本信息、手术名称以及手术知情同意书的签署情况。）

（The nurse checks the patient's basic information，the

name of the operation, and the signature of the informed consent.)

护士：请问您知道您今天要做什么手术吗？

N：Do you know what surgery you are going to receive today?

患者：做肝脏的，栓塞。

P：Liver operation, embolization.

护士：好的，是肝脏动脉化疗栓塞术。请问您是第一次做这个手术吗？

N：OK. It's hepatic arterial chemoembolization. Is this the first time you receive such an operation?

患者：对的。请问这个手术时间长吗？

P：Yes. How long will it take?

护士：这个手术时间不是很长，一般情况下大概 30 分钟。

N：Not very long, it takes about 30 minutes under normal circumstances.

患者：那这个手术是怎么做的？

P：What is the process?

护士：这个手术是从腹股沟处股动脉穿刺，利用专用的造影管沿着主动脉到右肝动脉，造影确定病变位置，然后局部用药，杀死不好的细胞。

N：The operation starts with a puncture of the femoral artery in the inguinal region, pushing a specialized catheter via aorta into the hepatic arteries to determine the location of the lesions by angiography, and then inject drugs to the local lesion area to eliminate abnormal cells.

患者：我需要麻醉吗？

P：Do I need anesthesia?

护士：需要的，但您的麻醉方式是局麻，整个过程中人都是清醒的。术中如果您有任何不适，都可以和我们讲。

N：Yes, but only local anesthesia is required. You will be conscious during the whole procedure, so you can tell us if you have any discomfort.

患者：好的，我明白了。谢谢护士。刚才我还有点紧张，现在好多了。

P：OK, I see. Thank you. I was a little nervous a moment ago, but now I feel much better.

护士：不用谢，应该的。请问您需要小便吗？

N：You are welcome. Do you need to go to urinate now?

患者：需要，你们这里有卫生间吗？

P：Yeah, where is the bathroom?

护士：有，我带您去。从这里直走，走到底向右转就是了。

N：I'll show you. Go straight ahead, and then turn right at the end of the corridor.

（患者从卫生间出来，来到手术等候区。）

(The patient comes out of the bathroom and goes to the surgical waiting area.)

护士：我们这里有 5 个手术间，您今天的手术在 1 号手术间进行。您现在是在手术等候区，一会儿会有人接您进去。每个手术间在进行手术时都会有射线，请您不要随意走动。有事可以随时问我，您现在休息下，等一下就轮到您了。

N：There are 5 surgical rooms. Your surgery will be performed at room number one. You are now in the surgical waiting area. We will escort you to the room later on. Because the radiation is used in the surgery, please do not walk around. We can help you if you need anything. Please have a rest now, you are next for the surgery.

患者：好的。

P：OK.

[Phrases]

under normal circumstances　　　　一般情况下

operating room	手术室
on duty	值班
basic information	基本信息

手术中

During the operation

[Glossary]

sterile drape	无菌巾单
hepatic arteriography	肝动脉造影
local anesthetic	局麻药
lidocaine	利多卡因
chemotherapy medicine	化疗药
epirubicin	表柔比星
hydroxycamptothecin（HCPT）	羟喜树碱
gelatin sponge particle	明胶海绵颗粒
gauze	纱布
compressor	压迫器

[Scenario]

（患者已经躺在手术床上，无菌单子已经铺好，手术材料准备完毕。）

（The patient is lying on the operating table. The sterile drape has been covered and the surgical materials are ready.）

护士：教授，手术材料已经准备好了。肝动脉造影导管、5F鞘、高压连接管、三通、造影导丝、注射器、酒精纱布都准备好了。

N：Professor，the operating materials are ready. Hepatic arteriography catheter，5F hemostasis，high-pressure connection catheter，three-way stopcock，angiographic guide wire，injector，and alcohol gauze are all prepared.

医生：好的，准备手术。

D：All right，let's start the surgery.

（再次核查患者的基本信息、手术名称及手术方式。）

（Recheck the patient's basic information，name and method of the operation.）

医生：局麻药利多卡因 5 ml。

D：Local anesthetic，lidocaine，5 ml.

护士：好的，局麻药，利多卡因 5 ml，请核对。

N：All right，local anesthetic，lidocaine，5 ml，please check.

（医生给患者股动脉穿刺成功，造影管已经到位，准备造影。）

（The doctor successfully punctured the femoral artery，placed the catheter in the right position and is ready to inject the contrast.）

医生：接下来准备造影，护士可以准备化疗药物了。

D：Now we are going to do angiography. Please prepare the chemotherapy medicine.

护士：好的。

N：OK.

（造影结束，已经确定病变部位。）

（The lesion site has been identified and confirmed by the angiogram.）

医生：现在需要配化疗药。表柔比星 20 mg + 20 ml 0.9% 氯化钠，羟喜树碱 20 mg + 20 ml 0.9% 氯化钠。

D：Now we need the medicine. Epirubicin 20 mg + 20 ml 0.9% NS，HCPT 20 mg + 20 ml 0.9% NS.

护士：好的，表柔比星 20 mg + 20 ml 0.9% 氯化钠，羟喜树碱 20 mg + 20 ml 0.9% 氯化钠。

N：All right. Epirubicin 20 mg + 20 ml 0.9% NS，HCPT 20 mg + 20 ml 0.9% NS.

护士：教授，药已经配好了，需要现在给您吗？

N：Professor, the medicine is ready. Do you need it now?

医生：对的。

D：Yes.

护士：表柔比星 20 mg + 20 ml 0.9% 氯化钠，羟喜树碱 20 mg + 20 ml 0.9% 氯化钠。请核对。

N：Epirubicin 20 mg + 20 ml 0.9% NS, HCPT 20 mg + 20 ml 0.9% NS. Check, please.

医生：好的。现在还需要明胶海绵颗粒。

D：All right. Gelatin sponge particles are also needed.

护士：请问教授，明胶海绵颗粒需要多大型号？

N：Professor, what size please?

医生：型号：350 - 560。

D：Size：350 - 560.

护士：好的。350 - 560 的明胶海绵颗粒一瓶。请核对。

N：OK, 350 - 560 gelatin sponge particles, one bottle. Check, please.

医生：手术结束了。

D：The operation is done.

护士：好的，纱布和压迫器已准备完毕。

N：OK. Gauze and compressor are ready.

[Phrases]

operating table	手术台
operating material	手术材料
be identified	被识别

手术后
After the operation

[Glossary]

gastrointestinal response	胃肠道反应
throw up	呕吐

choking	哽塞
asphyxia	窒息
antiemetic	止吐剂；止吐的
femoral artery	股动脉
pressure bandaging	加压包扎
sandbag compression	沙袋压迫
thrombosis	血栓形成
handheld urinal	尿壶
bedpan	便盆

[Scenario]

护士：张建，手术做好了，现在感觉怎么样？

N: Mr. Zhang, the operation is finished. How are you doing now?

患者：现在还可以，稍微有点恶心。

P: Not bad，but just a little disgusted.

护士：这个是用药之后最常见的胃肠道反应。如果您想呕吐，头偏向一侧，以免误吸引起呛咳或窒息。一般术后 3～4 天胃肠道反应基本消失。呕吐后，可以喝点温水漱口，到病房后，更换干净的衣服。如果呕吐严重，医生会给您开止吐的药物。

N: This is the most common gastrointestinal side effect after the medication. If you want to throw up, turn your head to one side to prevent choking or asphyxia. Most gastrointestinal side effect will disappear 3～4 days after the surgery. After vomiting, you can drink some warm water to rinse your mouth. You may change some clean clothes after arriving at the ward. If vomiting is severe，the doctor will prescribe antiemetic drugs for you.

患者：我晚饭可以吃点什么？

P: What can I have for supper?

护士：术后 2 小时，如果没有呕吐，可以吃点清淡、易消化
的食物，像稀饭、面条、麦片等。不能吃油煎和刺激
性的食物。

N：If there is no vomiting within 2 hours after the
surgery, you can eat some light and digestible foods,
such as congee, noodles, oatmeal and so on. Do not
eat fried and spicy foods.

患者：我什么时候可以下床活动？

P：When can I get off bed for a walk?

护士：24 小时后可以下地走路。您的手术穿刺的是股动
脉，术后需要平卧 24 小时，手术部位加压包扎，沙袋
压迫 6 小时。做手术那侧的腿保持伸直 12～24 小
时。可以左右平移，防止血栓形成。

N：You may take a walk 24 hours after the operation. As
a puncture was given to the femoral artery in your
operation, you will need to lie on your back for 24
hours after the surgery and the operating wound needs
pressure bandaging with sandbag compression for 6
hours. The operated leg should be kept straight for
12～24 hours. You are encouraged to move this leg
horizontally to prevent thrombosis.

患者：大小便怎么办？

P：What if I want to urinate or defecate?

护士：病房有尿壶和便盆，只能在床上大小便，以免引起股
动脉处压迫止血松动而大出血。术前病房护士已经
告诉你们要训练在床上大小便了吧？

N：There are handheld urinal and bedpan in the ward,
you should try to urinate and defecate in bed with
them to prevent bleeding from loss of femoral artery
pressure. I believe the ward nurse has instructed you
on training yourself to excrete on the bed before the
operation.

患者：是的。

P：Yes.

护士：现在马上送您回病房，您的鞋子和衣服已经放在车子下面的篮子里了。祝您早日康复。

N：Now we are about to send you back to the ward. We have put your shoes and clothes in the basket below the gurney. I wish you a speedy recovery.

患者：谢谢。

P：Thank you.

[Phrases]

gurney	轮床
a little disgusted	有点恶心
spicy food	刺激性食物
bleeding	出血

17. Health Education for Patients Undergoing Liver Biopsy
肝穿刺活检术患者的健康教育

[Glossary]

biopsy	活检
ultrasound	超声
sweat	出汗
deviation	偏离
pathological	病理的

[Scenario]

护士：张丹，您好，明天您要做肝穿刺活检，现在给您讲解一些肝穿刺活检的相关知识。

N：Hello，Zhang Dan. Tomorrow you're going to have a liver biopsy. Now I'll tell you some details about it.

患者：好的。

P：Good.

护士：肝穿刺活检是在 B 超、CT 引导下进行穿刺，从而获取病理资料。手术前需要禁食 4 小时，手术回来 2 小时后可进软食，禁食辛辣刺激、生冷的食物，需要平卧 6～8 小时。手术回来后会有轻微疼痛、出汗。如果疼痛加剧或有其他的不适，及时告知我们，我们会给您及时处理的。

N：The liver biopsy is performed with a puncture needle guided by ultrasound or CT to obtain pathological sample. Before the surgery you need to fast for 4 hours，and you may eat some soft foods 2 hours after the surgery，but do not eat spicy or cold foods. You should stay in bed for 6～8 hours after the surgery.

You will feel slight pain or sweat. If the pain worsens or other discomfort occurs，just tell us timely. We'll take care of it in time.

患者：好的，我明白了，但我还是有点紧张，怎么办？手术伤口大吗？

P：OK，I see，but I'm still a little nervous. What should I do? Is the size of surgical wound big?

护士：您的手术是局部麻醉的，手术后的伤口只有针尖大，因此您不用那么紧张。回来后我们还会继续观察您的伤口有无渗血、渗液的，不用担心。

N：The surgery is performed under local anesthesia，and the wound size is only as small as a pinpoint，so you do not have to be so nervous. When you come back，we will continue to observe whether your wound is bleeding or has discharge. Take it easy.

患者：手术过程中我要注意什么吗？

P：What should I pay attention to during the surgery?

护士：术中需要屏气，因为呼吸、咳嗽会导致穿刺针偏离，造成不良的后果。现在您需要放松身体，保证夜间有良好的睡眠。

N：You need to hold your breath during the biopsy because breathing or coughing can lead to deviation of the biopsy needle from the lesion. It may cause unwanted consequences. For now，you need to relax and have a good night's sleep.

患者：我会积极配合医生的，病理报告大概需要多长时间？

P：I'll try my best to cooperate with the doctor. How long will I have my pathology result?

护士：最快需要 7 天。

N：At least 7 days.

患者：要一周这么久！我能先出院吗？

P：A week is too long for me. Can I be discharged before

I get the pathology result?

护士：请和您的医生沟通一下。一般可以先回家，等病理
　　　报告出来后，您的医生会把结果告诉您，便于您考虑
　　　后续的治疗。

N：Please consult your doctor. Usually you can wait the
　　pathology result at your home. Your doctor will
　　contact you and discuss the treatment plan with you
　　after the result is out.

患者：好的。谢谢您。

P：All right. Thank you very much.

[**Phrases**]

slight pain	轻度疼痛
local anesthesia	局部麻醉
pay attention to	注意
cooperate with	与……合作
hold the breath	屏气
lead to	导致
puncture needle	穿刺针

Nursing Care of the Use and Observation of Antineoplastic Drugs

抗肿瘤药物使用与观察的护理

1. Health Education for Patients with Arsenic Trioxide Chemotherapy Treatment
三氧化二砷静脉化疗患者的健康教育

[Glossary]

intravenous chemotherapy	静脉化疗
arsenic trioxide	三氧化二砷
side effect	副作用;不良反应
nausea	恶心
intravenous extravasation	液体外渗
gastrointestinal reaction	胃肠道反应
drip rate	滴速
cross infection	交叉感染

[Scenario]

护士：李先生，您好，我是您的责任护士李阳。根据医嘱，明天即将为您进行三氧化二砷静脉化疗治疗，请问您有什么疑问吗？

N：How are you? Mr. Li. I am your primary nurse. My name is Li Yang. According to the doctor's order, you will receive intravenous chemotherapy treatment with arsenic trioxide tomorrow. Do you have any questions about this treatment?

患者：李护士，我想了解一下三氧化二砷是什么药品，用药以后会有哪些不良反应。

P：Nurse Li, I would like to know more about arsenic trioxide. Are there any side effects of this medicine?

护士：三氧化二砷，俗称砒霜，对肝癌细胞株具有明显的生长抑制作用，但它也有可能会引起恶心、呕吐、厌食、腹痛、腹泻、体重减轻、颜面水肿等常见的不良反应。

不过不要过于紧张,我们会对症处理,并且这些症状一般在停药后都会消失。

N：Arsenic trioxide is commonly known as arsenic. It has significant inhibitory effects on the growth of liver cancer cells. The common side effects are nausea, vomiting, anorexia, abdominal pain, diarrhea, weight loss, facial bloating and others. But do not be too nervous. We will give medicine to deal with the side effects and they usually subside or disappear after the chemotherapy.

患者：护士,那我还需要注意些什么吗?

P：Nurse, what else do I have to pay attention to?

护士：液体会通过静脉滴注的途径来进行,所以我会为您留置一根中心静脉导管,以确保药物的有效使用,同时也可以避免因外周静脉留置引起的液体外渗等情况发生。

N：You will be treated via intravenous drip through the central venous catheter. We will place a central venous catheter in your body to ensure the effectiveness of drugs and to avoid intravenous extravasation by peripheral venous indwelling.

患者：好的,知道了。

P：OK，I see.

护士：因为在使用完药物后可能会出现恶心、呕吐、厌食等情况,所以我建议您治疗当日提前进食早餐。我们会在进食 3～4 小时后再进行治疗,这样就可有效缓解胃肠道反应。治疗期每日饮水量需在 2 500 ml 以上,并多饮用富含维生素 C 的果汁。忌食煎炸、油腻等刺激性食物,宜少食多餐,多吃清淡可口、易消化、富含蛋白质、铁和维生素的食物。

N：Because you may have symptoms like nausea, vomiting, anorexia after the use of drugs, I suggest that you should eat breakfast earlier on the day of treatment. The treatment will start 3~4 hours after the breakfast, so that the gastrointestinal reactions can be effectively relieved. During the treatment, you should drink more than 2 500 ml water every day. Besides, please drink more juice which contains rich vitamin C. Don't eat irritant foods like fried and greasy ones. Eat less but more often a day, and light, tasty, digestible, protein-rich, iron-rich and vitamin-rich foods are recommended.

患者：好的。

P：OK.

护士：根据药物使用的要求，需要静滴 3～4 小时，所以您不可以随意调节滴速。

N：According to the instructions of the drug, it will take 3~4 hours to complete the drip, so don't adjust the drip rate by yourself.

患者：这么长时间！那还有其他要注意的吗？

P：It's such a long time! What else do I have to pay attention to?

护士：在治疗的第 7 天后可能会出现不同程度的眼睑水肿，那时我们会限制您的钠盐及饮水量的摄入，必要时您可以垫高枕头来缓解水肿。我们也会每日观察您体重及尿量的变化。这段时间，请以卧床休息为主，适当进行床边活动。您还需要关注您的大小便颜色及皮肤、巩膜的颜色，注意保护皮肤，防止因瘙痒而抓破皮。

N：In addition, variable degrees of eyelid edema may occur after seven days' treatment. If this happens your sodium and water intake will be restricted. You may also use high pillow to reduce the edema. We will observe and record your daily body weight and urine output carefully. During this period you should have a good rest and moderate exercises at bedside. You should also pay attention to the color of your urine, feces, skin as well as sclera. Please protect your skin to prevent scratching the wound due to itchiness.

患者: 好的。

P: Got it.

护士: 平时要注意休息,增强免疫力。减少外出,防止感冒或交叉感染。

N: You should have a good rest and therefore enhance your immunity. You should also limit your time of going out in order to prevent getting a cold or other cross infections.

患者: 好的,我会的。谢谢您!

P: OK, I will. Thank you!

[Phrases]

enhance immunity	增强免疫力
due to	由于
irritant food	刺激性食物
greasy food	油腻的食物
central venous	中心静脉的
be commonly known as	俗称
be too nervous	过于紧张

2. Application and Observation of Cisplatin
   顺铂的使用与观察

[Glossary]

cisplatin	顺铂
ovarian	卵巢的
cervical	子宫颈的
endometrial	子宫内膜的
prostate	前列腺
melanoma	黑色素瘤
sarcoma	肉瘤
malignant	恶性的
lymphoma	淋巴瘤
ototoxicity	耳毒性

[Scenario]

患者：李护士，能咨询你一些问题吗？

P：Nurse Li, can I ask you some questions?

护士：当然可以，张叔叔，您有什么问题？

N：Sure, Mr. Zhang, what do you want to know?

患者：我想了解一下顺铂这个药物的一些信息。

P：I would like to know more details about cisplatin.

护士：是医生已经确定您的方案了吗？您是想了解这个药的作用吧？

N：Has the doctor already decided your treatment plan? Do you want to know the effect of this medicine?

患者：医生给我推荐了几个方案，我想都了解一下。

P：The doctor recommended me several treatment options, and I want to know their advantages and disadvantages.

护士：好的，顺铂适用于小细胞与非小细胞肺癌、睾丸癌、
　　　卵巢癌、宫颈癌、子宫内膜癌、前列腺癌、膀胱癌、黑
　　　色素瘤、肉瘤、头颈部肿瘤及各种鳞状上皮癌和恶性
　　　淋巴瘤的治疗。

N：All right，cisplatin is a chemotherapy medicine
　　commonly used in the treatment of small cell lung
　　cancer，non-small cell lung cancer，testicular cancer，
　　ovarian cancer，cervical cancer，endometrial cancer，
　　prostate cancer，bladder cancer，melanoma，
　　sarcoma，tumors of the head and neck，various types
　　of squamous cell carcinoma，and malignant lymphoma.

患者：这个药应用还是很广的，怎么用这个药？是静脉
　　　滴吗？

P：It seems that this drug is widely used. How do you use
　　this medicine? By intravenous infusion?

护士：静脉滴注或动脉注射都可以，一般是根据患者的体
　　　表面积计算剂量，连用5日，间隔2周可重复用药。

N：Intravenous infusion or arterial injection can be used.
　　We calculate the dosage based on patients' body
　　surface area. The patient is usually treated 5 days
　　consecutively as a session and the treatment session can
　　be repeated after a two weeks' interval.

患者：这个药有什么不良反应？

P：What are the adverse effects of this medicine?

护士：最常见的不良反应为胃肠道反应，例如腹泻、恶心、
　　　呕吐及黏膜炎。此外，还包括中性粒细胞减少、血小
　　　板减少、耳毒性以及肾脏毒性。

N：The most common side effects are gastrointestinal
　　symptoms such as diarrhea，nausea，vomiting and
　　mucositis. Other side effects include neutropenia，
　　thrombocytopenia，ototoxicity and renal toxicity.

患者：那我还需要注意点什么？

P: What else do I need to pay attention to?

护士: 最重要的是多喝水, 就是我们说的大量输液水化疗法。建议每日饮水 2 500~3 000 ml, 这样可以降低肾脏毒性反应。此外, 您还需要关注穿刺处的局部情况。

N: The most important thing you should do is to drink a lot of water. We call it hydration therapy. We advise our patients to drink 2 500 to 3 000 ml water daily. This will reduce the kidney toxicity of cisplatin. In addition, you should pay attention to the injection site.

患者: 好的, 我心里有数了。

P: Okay, I got it.

护士: 您还需要了解些什么?

N: Anything else do you want to know?

患者: 我想到再问你。

P: Not now. I will ask if anything is coming to my mind.

护士: 好的。

N: No problem.

[Phrases]

small cell lung cancer	小细胞肺癌
non-small cell lung cancer	非小细胞肺癌
testicular cancer	睾丸癌
bladder cancer	膀胱癌
squamous cell	鳞状细胞
arterial injection	动脉注射
body surface area	体表面积
renal toxicity	肾毒性

3. Application and Observation of Epirubicin
　　表柔比星的使用与观察

[Glossary]

epirubicin	表柔比星
wristband	腕带
anthracycline	蒽环类
antibiotic	抗生素
replication	复制
mechanism	机制
reversible	可逆的
inhibit	抑制

[Scenario]

护士：徐伯伯，让我看一下您的腕带。

N：Mr. Xu, may I see your wristband please?

患者：我戴着好好的。

P：It is fine.

护士：我需要核对一下您的信息。现在要给您静滴表柔比星，请问您叫什么名字？

N：I need to check your information. Now I will give you an intravenous infusion of epirubicin. Your name please?

患者：我叫徐圣。

P：My name is Xu Sheng.

护士：为了您的用药安全，我还是得确认一下，您知道这个药的作用吗？

N：I just want to double check if you know why your doctor uses this medicine.

患者：不知道具体作用，只知道是治疗我这个疾病的，我相信医生。

P：I don't know the specific effect of this medicine except I was told it is used for my condition. I trust my doctor.

护士：好的，我给您普及一下。

N：OK，I'll give you some introduction about this medicine.

患者：非常感谢！

P：Thank you very much!

护士：表柔比星又叫法玛新，属蒽环类抗生素，通过干扰肿瘤细胞的 DNA 复制来抑制其生长。

N：Epirubicin，also known as pharmorubicin，is an anthracycline antibiotic. It inhibits the growth of cancer cells by interfering its DNA replication.

患者：我好像听不懂。

P：I do not understand what you have said.

护士：这是作用机制，您了解一下就可以了。

N：This is the mechanism how the drug works. It just gives you a general idea of this medicine.

患者：好的。

P：OK.

护士：我来说说副作用。这个药用过之后可能会出现呕吐、高热、脱发。脱发占病例中 60%～90%，一般可逆。用药后 1～2 天可能出现尿液红染，5～10 天可能出现黏膜炎，10～14 天可能出现中性粒细胞减少，这些症状都是正常的药物反应。

N：Now let's talk about the side effects of this medicine. The most common side effects are vomiting，high fever and alopecia. The alopecia occurs in 60% to 90% of the patients，and it is reversible. Your urine may appear reddish 1 to 2 days after the treatment；mucosa inflammation may occur 5 to 10 days after the treatment；and neutropenia may occur 10 to 14 days after the treatment. These side effects are expected and are not unusual.

患者：嗯。

P：I see.

护士：治疗结束后，我们会定期给您复查血象，来观察您身体的一些变化。

N：We will do routine check-up and blood work on you at a regular basis after the treatment.

患者：好的。

P：All right.

护士：还会通过心电图来检查您的心脏功能。

N：We will also check on your heart function by ECG.

患者：我知道了。

P：OK，I see.

护士：我会观察您用药后的反应，并及时汇报医生，给予相应的处理。

N：I will keep my eye on your response to the medicine and communicate with your doctor promptly so that your doctor will give you follow-up treatment accordingly when it is necessary.

患者：谢谢。

P：Thank you.

[Phrases]

side effect	副作用
high fever	高热
alopecia	脱发
neutropenia	中性粒细胞减少

4. Application and Observation of Docetaxel
　　多西他赛的使用与观察

[Glossary]

docetaxel	多西他赛
chemotherapy	化疗
metastatic	转移性的
bone marrow	骨髓
gastrointestinal	胃肠道的
neurotoxicity	神经毒性
cardiovascular	心血管的
hypotension	低血压
itchiness	瘙痒
aseptic	无菌的

[Scenario]

护士 1：吴教员，今天 3 床曾阿姨静滴多西他赛，我巡视的时候她询问了我这个药物的相关知识，我不是很清楚，您能给我讲讲吗？我想一会去给患者讲解。

N1：Teacher Wu, Ms. Zeng in bed 3 was treated with docetaxel intravenously. Today she asked me about this medicine when I visited her. I don't know a lot. Could you please tell me about it? I would like to explain it to the patient a moment later.

护士 2：小芳，你是实习同学，对这个药物不了解很正常。3 床阿姨我给她讲过一次了，可能她忘了，又询问你，一会我们一起再给患者做一次药物宣教。

N2：Xiao Fang, no worries. I understand that you do not know about this drug as you are an intern. The patient may have forgotten the instruction I gave to her before. We can do that again together.

护士 1：好的。

N1：All right.

护士 2：这是一个化疗药物，主要适用于以顺铂为主的化疗失败的晚期及转移性非小细胞肺癌或转移性乳腺癌的患者。用法为静脉滴注。这个药用之前需要服用糖皮质激素 3 天，以防出现过敏反应和体液潴留。

N2：This chemotherapy drug is mainly used for patients with advanced or metastatic non-small cell lung carcinoma and metastatic breast cancers that have failed to respond to cisplatin. It is administered via intravenous drip. The patient needs to receive corticosteroids for 3 days before taking docetaxel in order to prevent allergies and fluid retention.

护士 1：不良反应有哪些？

N1：What are the side effects?

护士 2：不良反应有：过敏反应、体液潴留、骨髓抑制、神经毒性反应、胃肠道反应、心血管副反应、皮肤反应等，严重者有低血压与支气管痉挛，需中断治疗。而皮肤反应主要表现为红斑，常见于手足，有时伴有瘙痒。

N2：The side effects include allergic reactions, fluid retention, bone marrow suppression, neurotoxicity, gastrointestinal reactions, cardiovascular adverse reactions, skin reactions or hypotension and bronchial spasm in severe cases. If any of these happen, we need to stop the treatment. The allergic skin reaction includes rash and itchiness commonly found in the hands and feet.

护士 1：不良反应真多，我有点记不住了。

N1：It has so many adverse reactions that I cannot

memorize all of them.

护士2：你可以这样记忆，如皮肤的反应、呼吸系统的、消化系统的、循环系统的等。

N2：You can memorize them according to tissue systems, such as skin reactions, respiratory system, digestive system, circulatory system, and so on.

护士1：这样好像也没有那么难了。

N1：Oh, it doesn't seem so difficult now.

护士2：我们要重点注意以下几点：当医生要使用这个药物时要查看医生是否开激素，激素会增加体液潴留的发生，要随时观察患者的体重变化；在滴注药物前，要做到现配现用；静滴几分钟后可能发生过敏反应，应注意观察患者的生命体征变化，准备好相应的急救设施；我们还要做好手卫生，做到无菌操作。

N2：We have to pay particular attention to several things: we need to check if the doctor has prescribed corticosteroid before the treatment. As corticosteroid can increase the morbidity of body fluid retention, we need to observe the patient's weight changes during the treatment. The drug should be prepared few minutes right before using. Remember to monitor the allergic reactions and vital signs during the administration, and have plans to deal with the side effects when it is needed. Also, we have to keep our hands clean and follow aseptic operation protocols.

护士1：我知道了。

N1：OK, I see.

护士2：其实还有很多地方需要我们注意，比如说做好患者的心理护理，这个也非常重要。

N2：In fact, there are a lot of other things we must pay

attention to，for example，the patient's psychological care.

护士 1：教员，我记住了，我会好好学习的。

N1：I will keep these in mind and study hard later.

护士 2：很好。

N2：Very good.

［Phrases］

intern	实习生
breast cancer	乳腺癌
in order to	为了
fluid retention	体液潴留
adverse reaction	不良反应
allergic reaction	过敏反应
bronchial spasm	支气管痉挛
respiratory system	呼吸系统
digestive system	消化系统
circulatory system	循环系统

5. Application and Observation of Fluorouracil
   氟尿嘧啶的使用与观察

[Glossary]

fluorouracil	氟尿嘧啶
precaution	预防措施;注意事项
oropharyngeal	口咽部
inevitably	不可避免地
pigmentation	色素沉着
vulnerable	脆弱的
white blood cell	白细胞

[Scenario]

护士:张阿姨,从今天开始您需要氟尿嘧啶治疗了,在使用这个药物之前我需要告知您这个药物的不良反应和注意事项。

N:Ms. Zhang, you will have a fluorouracil treatment from today. Let's talk about the side effects and precautions we have to take.

患者:好的。

P:Good.

护士:这个药用过之后最有可能会出现恶心、呕吐等胃肠道反应,严重时可出现口咽部及肠道溃疡。

N:You may have nausea, vomiting and other gastrointestinal reactions after the treatment. In severe cases, oropharyngeal ulcer and intestinal ulcer may occur.

患者:我有点担心,估计会非常难受吧。

P:I am worried about the side effects of the treatment. It must be very uncomfortable.

护士：张阿姨,使用这类特殊药物难免会有一些副作用,我
　　　们提前告知您,是为了在使用的过程中减少不必要
　　　的紧张。其实,我们医生会根据您的情况给予预防,
　　　让这些反应尽可能不发生或者减少药物对您的
　　　伤害。

N：Ms. Zhang, this kind of special drugs will inevitably
　　have some side effects. The aim we inform you in
　　advance is to make you feel less nervous during the
　　treatment. In fact, your doctor may give you some
　　medicine according to your situation to prevent or
　　reduce the side effects.

患者：那就好,还有什么其他的副作用?

P：That's good. Are there any other side effects?

护士：治疗后可能出现皮肤色素沉着、脱发等,您看到这些
　　　不要紧张。

N：Skin pigmentation and hair loss are the common side
　　effects after the treatment. Please be aware of that.

患者：嗯,其他患者跟我说过,这个我不担心。

P：Well, other patients have told me these side effects, I
　　don't worry about them.

护士：在用药后还有可能会出现白细胞下降,所以我们会
　　　定期给您复查血常规。

N：Your white blood cell count may decrease after the
　　chemotherapy, so we'll check it on a regular basis.

患者：好的。

P：All right.

护士：如果您的白细胞数量太少,代表免疫系统非常脆弱,
　　　您要注意保暖,不要受寒,经常开窗通风,不要去人
　　　流密集的地方,避免感染。医生会给予药物,增加白
　　　细胞数量。

N：Your immunity will become vulnerable if your white
　　blood cell count is significantly reduced after the

chemotherapy. We would like to remind you to keep warm to avoid catching a cold. Moreover, to reduce the chance of infection, please open the window more often for good air ventilation, and try not to go to crowded places. The doctor will also prescribe some medicine to get your white blood cell count back to normal.

患者：好的，谢谢。

P: OK, thank you.

[Phrases]

in advance	预先
in fact	事实上
according to	根据
keep warm	保暖
crowded place	人流密集的地方

6. Application and Observation of Irinotecan
伊立替康的使用与观察

[Glossary]

irinotecan	伊利替康
prescribe	开处方
precaution	注意事项
antidiarrheal	止泻剂
neutropenia	中性粒细胞减少
fatigue	疲乏

[Scenario]

护士：李叔叔，您好！我是您的责任护士李双。

N：Hello! Mr. Li! I'm your primary nurse. My name is Li Shuang.

患者：您好。

P：Oh，hello!

护士：现在感觉怎么样？

N：How do you feel now?

患者：挺好的。

P：I am fine.

护士：今天医生给您开了伊立替康，现在我给您说一下其不良反应和注意事项。

N：The doctor prescribed irinotecan for you today. Now I'll tell you something about the side effects and precautions of taking this medicine.

患者：好的。

P：All right.

护士：用药 24 小时后可能会出现迟发性腹泻，当您出现反应的时候不要紧张，只要及时补充液体，同时配合使用止泻药，就不会对您的身体造成伤害。

N：Delayed diarrhea may occur 24 hours after the treatment. But don't be nervous when you have this reaction. We will give you fluid replacement as well as antidiarrheal drugs in time, it will not do harm to your health.

患者：好的。

P：OK.

护士：部分患者可能会出现恶心、呕吐等胃肠道反应，如反应严重，医生会使用止吐药物。

N：Some patients may have gastrointestinal reactions like nausea and vomiting. If the reaction is serious, the doctor will use antiemetic drugs.

患者：我知道了。

P：I see.

护士：部分患者在用药后还会出现中性粒细胞减少合并发热，所以我们会定期给您测量体温，复查血常规。

N：As some patients may also have neutropenia and fever after the medication, we will measure your temperature and check your blood routine regularly.

患者：好的。

P：OK.

护士：部分患者用药后还会出现乏力、脱发等反应。

N：Some patients will experience fatigue, hair loss and other reactions after the medication.

患者：脱发厉害吗？

P：Is the hair loss serious?

护士：虽然会脱发，但是是可逆的，停药后头发会慢慢长出来。

N：Although your hair may fall off, it is reversible. They will slowly grow back after stopping taking the medicine.

患者：好的。

P：That's good.

护士：用药过程中有什么不舒服都可以来找我，我们会针
　　　对性地给您用药的。

N：Please let me know if you have any discomfort during
　　the treatment，so we will deal with it.

患者：好的，谢谢。

P：OK，thanks.

[Phrases]

delayed diarrhea	迟发性腹泻
fluid replacement	补液
do harm to	引起损害
antiemetic drug	止吐药
blood routine	血常规

Health Education of
Various Types of Catheter Care

各类导管护理的健康教育

1. Health Education for Patients Before Percutaneous Transhepatic Cholangiodrainage
经皮肝穿刺胆道引流术前患者的健康教育

[Glossary]

percutaneous	经皮的
transhepatic	肝穿刺
cholangiodrainage	胆道引流
bilirubin	胆红素
bile	胆汁
jaundice	黄疸
hepatoprotective	保肝的
decompression	解压
inflammation	炎症
endanger	危及

[Scenario]

护士：您好！请问是张力先生吗？我是您的责任护士孙芊。

N：Hello! Are you Zhang Li? I am your primary nurse. My name is Sun Qian.

患者：我是，有什么事情吗？

P：Yes, I am. What's the matter?

护士：今天您要在 DSA 下行 PTCD 术，也就是经皮肝穿刺胆道引流。由于您的胆红素高，需要通过这个手术来引流胆汁。

N：Today you are going to do a PTCD under DSA, which is percutaneous transhepatic cholangiodrainage. Because of your high bilirubin level, you need to receive this surgery to drain the bile.

患者：不能静滴一些保肝药物来治疗吗？为什么一定要
　　　引流？

P：Can it be treated with some hepatoprotective drugs intravenously? Why must I take this drainage operation?

护士：根据您现在的病情，这是对您最有效的治疗方案，输
　　　液已经不能解决您的重症黄疸，需减压引流。其实
　　　引流只是一种方式，不要紧张，就是在体内留置外引
　　　流管，把您体内过多的胆汁引流，以免引发炎症反应
　　　及系统性不良反应，甚至危及您的生命。

N：At this moment, the decompression drainage is the most effective treatment for your current condition, because infusion treatment is no longer useful to your severe jaundice. Don't worry. The decompression drainage treatment is actually just a method to reduce your jaundice. A drainage tube will be retained inside your body to drain out the bile continuously out of your body. That will prevent inflammation and systemic adverse reactions which may endanger your life.

患者：这么严重？

P：So serious?

护士：是的，所以您必须重视，但也不用过分紧张，一旦引
　　　流通畅，您的症状就会得到有效的缓解。

N：Yes, you must take this matter seriously, but there is no need to be overstrained. Once the drainage is successful, your symptoms will be alleviated effectively.

患者：好的，孙护士，我会配合医生治疗的。

P：OK, Nurse Sun, I'll cooperate with the doctor.

[Phrases]

current condition　　　　　　　目前的状况

effective treatment　　　　　　有效的治疗

2. Health Education for Patients After Percutaneous Transhepatic Cholangiodrainage
经皮肝穿刺胆道引流术后患者的健康教育

[Glossary]

drainage	引流
properly	正确地
twist	扭曲
bloody	血性的
quantity	量
transparent	透明的

[Scenario]

护士：您已经完成了相关的术前检查，治疗前需要禁食、禁水 4 小时。现在请在病房休息，卫勤中心工作人员会准时过来接您去手术室。

N：You have completed the relevant preoperative examination. Please don't eat or drink 4 hours before the treatment. Now you can have a rest in the ward, then our medical staff from the service center will take you to the operating room on time.

患者：好的，谢谢。那我术后要如何维护这根引流导管呢？

P：OK，thanks. How to take care of this catheter after the operation?

护士：首先要妥善固定引流管，防止导管滑出。其次要保持引流通畅，不能扭曲，特别注意在翻身时不要挤压引流管。

N：Firstly，the drainage tube should be properly fixed to prevent it from sliding out. Secondly，do not twist the drainage tube and ensure its patency. Pay special attention not to squeeze the drainage tube when you turn your body over.

患者：那我需要观察引流液吗？

P: Do I need to observe the drainage fluid?

护士：要的。术后 24 小时内出现少量的血性引流液是正常情况。若发现大量的血性液体，说明可能出现了出血，应及时通知医生或者护士。每天要观察引流液的颜色、性质、量。正常的胆汁是金黄色透明的，每天的量在 500～1 000 ml。如果每天的量超过 1 000 ml 或引流量少，同时出现腹痛、发热、黄疸等症状，要及时报告医生或护士。如果每天的量很少，但是大便颜色是正常的，也不出现发热、腹痛、黄疸等症状，这也是正常的。

N：Yes. A small amount of blood-tinged drainage fluid within 24 hours after the operation is not unusual. If a large amount of bloody fluid is found, it means that hemorrhage may occur. You should inform the doctor or nurse as soon as possible. You need to observe the color, property and quantity of the drainage fluid every day. The normal bile should be golden and transparent with 500～1 000 ml of the daily amount. You should notify us in time if the daily bile amount exceeds 1 000 ml. You should alert us as well if the amount is too little and you have abdominal pain, fever or jaundice. It is considered a normal condition if the drainage fluid amount is relatively small but the color of the stool is fine and none of above symptoms occur.

患者：那我能起床活动吗？

P: Can I get up and do some exercises?

护士：可以的，起床后用别针把导管固定在同侧衣服上，保持引流袋的位置低于穿刺点，以防引流袋里的液体反流至胆管引起感染。

N：Sure. When you get up, you should fix the catheter on the same side of the clothes with a pin and keep the location of the drainage bag lower than the puncture point to prevent the infection caused by the reflux of the liquid in the drainage bag to the bile duct.

患者：我知道了，我能洗澡吗？

P：I got it. Can I take a shower?

护士：伤口敷料需要保持清洁干燥，洗澡容易污染穿刺口，最好擦浴。

N：You must keep the surgical dressing clean and dry, you'd better have sponge bath instead, because showering may contaminate your puncture site easily.

患者：我能吃些什么呢？

P：What can I eat?

护士：在早期，应该遵循少量多餐的原则，饮食以清淡、易消化的低脂流质为主。第1天先进食米汤、菜汁等，进食后密切观察有无腹胀、腹痛、恶心等不适；第2天可进食鱼汤、肉汤、稀饭、新鲜果汁等，观察2～3天，若仍无腹痛、腹胀等不适，3周以后再逐渐恢复每日三餐的正常饮食习惯。多进食富含维生素及优质蛋白的食物，同时多饮水，以利于冲洗尿中过量的胆盐淤积。

N：In the early stage, you should follow the principle of eating less but more often. The main diet should be light and digestible low-fat liquid. On the first day after the operation, you may take rice soup, vegetable juice, etc. , and observe whether you have abdominal distension, abdominal pain, nausea, etc. On the second day, you may have fish soup, broth, rice porridge and fresh fruit juice, etc. , observing for 2～3 days，make sure you feel good and have no abdominal pain or abdominal distension，then you may resume your normal eating habits of three meals a day gradually in 3 weeks. It is suggested to eat more vitamin-rich and protein-rich foods，and drink more water，which helps to flush the excess bile salt deposition in the urine.

患者：好的。

P：All right.

护士：15 天复查一次，引流袋一周更换 2 次。如出现伤口纱布脱落，应及时来门诊更换；出现导管滑出、堵塞或腹痛、发热、黄疸等，要及时来门诊复诊。

N：Reexamination is required every 15 days，and the drainage bag needs to be changed twice a week. If the gauzes fall off，you should go to the outpatient department for replacement right away. If the catheter is blocked or slides out，or you have abdominal pain，fever or jaundice，go to see the doctor.

患者：好的，谢谢你！

P：OK，thank you!

护士：不用谢！

N：You are welcome!

[Phrases]

service center	服务中心
operating room	手术室
slide out	滑脱
drainage fluid	引流液
drainage tube	引流管
in time	及时
the color of the stool	大便的颜色

abdominal pain	腹痛
get up	起床
on the same side	同一侧
puncture point	穿刺点
early stage	早期
follow the principle	遵守原则

3. Health Education for Patients Before Central Venous Catheterization via Peripheral Vein
经外周静脉置入中心静脉导管置管前患者的健康教育

[Glossary]

peripherally	经外周的
insert	插入
central	中心的
catheter	导管
puncture	穿刺
irritant	刺激性的
professional	专业的
elbow	肘部
dilute	稀释
complication	并发症
venipuncture	静脉穿刺
diameter	直径
junction	结合处

[Scenario]

护士：李先生，您好。我是您的责任护士李美。由于您的治疗需要长期输注刺激性药物，最好留置中心静脉置管，如 PICC。

N：Hello, Mr. Li. I am your primary nurse Li Mei. Because your treatment requires long-term infusion of irritant drugs, a central venous catheter such as PICC is suggested to be retained.

患者：什么是 PICC?

P：What is PICC?

护士：PICC 即经外周静脉置入中心静脉导管，是由专业护士在靠近肘窝和上臂一个大的外周静脉穿刺插管，使其导管尖端位于上腔静脉。插入过程是微创，经常可以在床边进行。

N：PICC is peripherally inserted central catheter. Its placement is operated by a professional nurse through a large peripheral vein puncture near the elbow and upper arm, and the tip of the catheter would be located at the superior vena cava. The operation is minimally invasive and it can usually be done at bedside.

患者：使用 PICC 这种导管安全吗？

P：Is it safe?

护士：这是一种非常安全的治疗方式。药物经 PICC 直接进入中心静脉，短时间内被迅速稀释，大大减少了对血管的损伤，也降低了并发症的风险。

N：It is a very safe treatment. The drug injected into the PICC is transfused directly into the central vein, therefore can be quickly diluted in short time. In this way the damage to the blood vessels and the risk of complications are reduced remarkably.

患者：穿刺 PICC 大概要花多少钱啊？是不是很贵？

P：How much does the puncture of PICC cost? Is it expensive?

护士：不同的 PICC 价格不一样，我们目前使用的是巴德 4F 导管，价格在 2 000 元左右。

N：The prices of different PICCs are various. We are currently using the Bard 4F catheter, it is about RMB 2 000.

患者：那不是很贵。我现在有点紧张，穿刺的时候会不会很疼啊？

P：Not very expensive. I'm a little nervous now. Is it

painful during the operation?

护士：穿刺 PICC 和一般的静脉穿刺没有太大的区别，只是穿刺点相对而言会大一点，但是我们在穿刺之前会给您局部麻醉，您不会有太疼的感觉，所以不要太紧张。

N：PICC puncture is quite similar to the usual venipuncture，while the wound of the PICC puncture is relatively larger. We will give you local anesthesia before the puncture，so you will not feel much pain. Just take it easy.

患者：穿刺的管子粗吗？

P：Is the puncture tube thick?

护士：PICC 导管直径 1.40 mm，总长度 60 cm。

N：PICC's diameter is 1.40 mm and the total length is 60 cm.

患者：这么长？那会插到什么地方？

P：That sounds quite long. How far will it go into?

护士：虽然管道有 60 cm，但是并非全部进入您的体内，而是根据您的个体情况确定插入的长度。一般导管会到达上腔静脉的中下段处，靠近上腔静脉与右心房交界处。

N：Although the catheter is 60 cm in length，it will not be inserted entirely into your body. The inserted distance will be set according to your personal situation. Generally，the catheter will reach the middle-lower-end of the superior vena cava，near the junction between the superior vena cava and the right atrium.

患者：好的，我明白了。谢谢你的详细讲解，我现在没有那么紧张了。

P：OK，I see. Thank you for the detailed explanation. I am not so nervous now.

护士：不用谢，这是我应该做的。

N：You are welcome. It is my duty.

[**Phrases**]

long-term infusion	长期输注
minimally invasive	微创
central vein	中心静脉
in a short time	短期内
local anesthesia	局部麻醉
take it easy	不要紧张
vena cava	腔静脉

4. Health Education for Patients After Central Venous Catheterization via Peripheral Vein 经外周静脉置入中心静脉导管置管后 患者的健康教育

[Glossary]

intact	完整的
heparin	肝素
erythema	红斑
swelling	肿胀

[Scenario]

护士：李先生，您的 PICC 导管已经穿刺成功了，您现在感觉怎么样？

N：Mr. Li, your PICC has been successfully inserted. How are you feeling now?

患者：还可以。留置 PICC 后我还应注意什么？

P：I'm fine. What should I pay attention to after inserting the PICC?

护士：携带 PICC 的患者可以从事一般性日常工作、家务劳动、体育锻炼，但需避免使用置管侧的手臂提过重的物体或抬高上举，不可以行持重锻炼。薄膜敷料应干燥、清洁、完好、贴壁，不要擅自撕下贴膜。若贴膜卷曲、松动或贴膜下有汗液时，及时请护士更换。每周定期更换贴膜、肝素帽和冲洗导管一次以上。您应注意观察伤口，如有红斑、肿胀、发热、疼痛、渗出等异常时，要及时告知医务人员。

N：Patients with PICC can engage in normal daily work, housework, and physical exercises, but should avoid carrying or lifting heavy objects with the involved arm and avoid weight-lifting exercises. The dressing should be dry, clean, intact and adhesive, and do not tear it off. If the dressing is curled, loose or sweat appears under the film, please tell the nurse in time to replace. The dressing should be replaced at least once a week, along with heparin cap replacement and catheter flushing. You should often observe the wound, if erythema, swelling, fever, pain, exudation and other abnormalities are found, you need to inform the medical staff promptly.

患者：可以带着这条导管洗澡吗？

P：Can I take a bath with this catheter?

护士：可以淋浴，但不能浴盆泡澡或洗桑拿。在淋浴前请先固定好导管，然后用保鲜膜在贴膜外缠绕 3 圈，将穿刺点上下 15 cm 的范围包裹严密，最后在上下边缘处用胶布固定，防止进水。淋浴后及时检查敷料，如有潮湿、进水，请护士及时更换。

N：You can take a shower, but do not take a bath or sauna. Before the shower, secure the catheter in proper position first, then wrap around the dressing with plastic wrap for 3 loops. In order to prevent water from streaming into the catheter, the area around the puncture site with a radius of 15 cm should be tightly wrapped. Please recheck the dressing right after the shower. If it is wet or damp, please reach out to your nurse for replacement timely.

患者：PICC 能保留多长时间？

P：How long can the PICC be retained?

护士：PICC 可以在体内长时间留置，最长可以达一年。

N：PICC can be retained in the body for a long time, up to a year.

患者：如果导管内有回血我应该怎样处理？

P：What should I do if there is blood in the catheter?

护士：残留在肝素帽或导管里的血液不会伤害您，但是它有可能会增加感染及导管堵塞的危险，所以如果发现导管内有血液，应尽快前往医院冲洗导管。

N：The blood remaining in the heparin cap or catheter will not hurt you, but it may increase the risk of infection and catheter blockage. If blood is found inside the catheter, you should go to hospital to flush the catheter as soon as possible.

患者：其他还有什么需要注意的吗?

P：What else do I need to pay attention to?

护士：妥善固定导管，禁止牵拉，以防导管断裂或脱出体外。门诊时务必携带维护手册。导管出现滑脱、破损时，请在靠近穿刺部位，将破裂或渗漏以上部位折起，并用胶布固定，然后立即到就近的医疗点。

N：You also need to secure the catheter properly, and do not pull the catheter to prevent it from breakage or slippage. Remember to bring your maintenance manual when visiting the doctor at the clinic. If the catheter slides out or is damaged, you should fold it up near the puncture site in upper section of broken or leaked part, and secure it with tape, then go to hospital immediately.

患者：好的，我大概明白了，谢谢你，有问题我再问你。

P：OK，I have a general idea now. Thank you. May I come to you if I have further questions?

护士：好的，有问题您及时给我们护士或者医生打电话。

N：Of course. If you have any questions, don't hesitate to call us or your doctors immediately.

[Phrases]

daily work　　　　　　　　　　日常工作

engage in	从事
physical exercise	体育锻炼
heavy object	重物
tear off	撕下
medical staff	医务人员
wrap around	缠绕
as soon as possible	尽快

5. Health Education for Patients with Indwelling Urinary Catheter
留置导尿管患者的健康教育

[Glossary]

colorless	无色的
transparent	透明的
turbid	浑浊的
crystalline	结晶的
bladder	膀胱

[Scenario]

护士：您好，张先生。我是您的责任护士小孙。

N：Hello! Mr. Zhang. I am your primary nurse. You can call me Xiao Sun.

患者：你好！小孙。

P：Hello! Xiao Sun.

护士：由于您 12 小时未解小便，感觉腹胀，根据医嘱要给您留置导尿管。

N：Because you have no urine output for up to 12 hours, and you have abdominal distention, we will insert an indwelling catheter for you according to the medical order.

患者：好的，能简单介绍一下这个导尿管的作用吗？

P：All right. Could you please give me a brief introduction about the purpose of this catheter?

护士：这根导管主要是引流尿液，解除尿潴留问题。

N：This catheter is mainly used to drain your urine and relieve urinary retention.

患者：好的，谢谢。那我怎么维护这个导管？

P：OK，thanks. How do I maintain this catheter?

护士：要妥善固定引流管，防止导管滑出。要保持引流通畅，不能扭曲，特别注意睡觉、翻身时不能压住引流管。

N：You should secure the drainage catheter to prevent it from sliding out. Please don't twist or press on the catheter when you sleep or turn over in order to keep it unobstructed.

患者：那我需要观察引流液吗？

P：Do I need to keep an eye on the drainage fluid?

护士：要的，正常尿液是无色、透明或淡黄色，正常尿量每天 1 500～2 000 ml。如果发现尿液混浊、沉淀、有结晶时，应及时告知医生或护理人员。

N：Yes. Normally the urine is colorless, transparent or pale yellow with a daily output of 1 500～2 000 ml. If urine is found to be turbid, sedimented and crystalline, you should inform the doctors or nurses in time.

患者：那我能起床活动吗？

P：Can I get up and do some exercises?

护士：可以的，起床后用别针把导管固定在同侧衣服上，但引流袋的位置要低，不能高于穿刺点，以防引流袋里的液体反流引起感染。

N：Yes. Please use the pin to secure the catheter on the same side of your clothes. In order to prevent infection resulted from urine reflux, the location of the drainage bag should be lower than the puncture point.

患者：我知道了。

P：OK, I got it.

护士：每日要多饮水，2 000～3 000 ml，增加内冲洗作用，减少尿路感染的机会，同时也可以预防尿路结石的形成。

N: You need to drink enough water, about 2 000～3 000 ml per day. It will flush the waste out and reduce the risk of urinary tract infection. It can also reduce the risk of stone formation.

患者: 什么时候可以拔管?

P: When can the catheter be pulled out?

护士: 您需要先训练膀胱反射功能,可采用间歇式夹管方式。夹闭导尿管,每 3～4 小时开放一次,使膀胱定时充盈和排空,促进膀胱功能恢复,病情稳定后就可拔管。

N: Before removing the catheter, intermittent clamping of the catheter can be used to train bladder reflex function. The catheter should be opened with the interval of 3～4 hours, so that the bladder can be regularly filled and emptied to promote the recovery of bladder function. After your condition becomes stable, the catheter can be pulled out.

患者: 好的,谢谢你!

P: OK, thank you!

护士: 不用谢!

N: You are welcome!

[Phrases]

urinary catheter	导尿管
drain urine	引流尿液
urinary retention	尿潴留
slide out	滑脱
drainage fluid	引流液
pale yellow	淡黄色
the location of	……的位置
urinary tract infection	尿路感染
reflex function	反射功能

6. Health Education for Patients Undergoing Endoscopic Nasobiliary Drainage
行经内镜鼻胆管引流术患者的健康教育

[Glossary]

endoscopic	内窥镜的
nasobiliary	鼻胆管
drainage	引流
retrograde	逆行
cholangiopancreatography	胰胆管造影术
esophagus	食管
pharynx	咽部
nostril	鼻孔
jaundice	黄疸
inflammation	炎症
electrocardiogram	心电图
morphine	吗啡

[Scenario]

护士：王芳，您好，我是您的责任护士孙芊，现在来通知您明天的手术。

N: Hello, Wang Fang. I am your primary nurse Sun Qian. I am here to inform you of the surgery tomorrow.

患者：好的。

P: OK.

护士：根据医嘱，您明天要行 ENBD 术，手术之后会留置一根鼻胆管。

N: According to the advice of your doctor, tomorrow you are going to have ENBD, and a nasobiliary tube will be left in your body after the surgery.

患者：请问这是个什么手术？

P：What kind of operation is this?

护士：经内镜鼻胆管引流术是最为常用的内镜胆道引流方法。它是在诊断性逆行胆管造影（ERCP）技术的基础上建立起来的。它采用一根细长的塑料管在内镜下经十二指肠乳头插入胆管中，另一端经十二指肠、胃、食管、咽等从鼻孔引出体外，建立胆汁的体外引流途径。

N：Endoscopic nasobiliary drainage（ENBD）is the most commonly used endoscopic biliary drainage method. It is established on the basis of endoscopic retrograde cholangiopancreatography（ERCP）. By using this method a long plastic tube is inserted into the bile duct under the endoscope through the duodenal papilla，while the other end of the tube passes the duodenum，stomach，esophagus，pharynx and the nostril to estab-lish a pathway for bile drainage.

患者：有什么目的吗？

P：What is the purpose?

护士：ENBD 是简便有效的解除胆道梗阻的方法，通过引流达到减压、减黄、消炎的目的。

N：ENBD is a simple and effective way to alleviate biliary obstruction and to achieve the aim of decompression，eliminating jaundice and inflammation.

患者：那我术前需要准备什么吗？

P：What do I need to do before the surgery?

护士：胸片、心电图、血常规、血淀粉酶、出凝血时间等检查完善好。术日前禁食 12 小时、禁水 8 小时。年老、体弱及病情较重的患者可酌情补液支持。术前肌肉注射吗啡 50 mg，抑制胃肠蠕动，放松 Oddi 氏括约肌。

N：You need to complete the tests including chest X-ray, electrocardiogram, blood routine, blood amylase, clotting time before the operation. It requires fasting for 12 hours and no drinking for 8 hours before the surgery. For those elderly, fragile and seriously ill patients, fluid infusion can be used. Preoperative intramuscular injection of 50 mg of morphine is commonly provided to inhibit gastrointestinal peristalsis and relax Oddi sphincter.

患者：那术后呢？

P：What do I need to do after the surgery?

护士：一般术后禁食 24 小时，卧床休息，注意有无腹痛、腹胀、恶心、呕吐等情况，如有不适，报告医生处理。术后 3 小时及次晨分别查血、尿淀粉酶。

N：Under normal circumstances, you must fast for 24 hours and rest in bed. Pay attention to symptoms like abdominal pain, abdominal distension, nausea, vomiting, etc. If you feel uncomfortable, just tell the doctor. The blood and urine amylase should be analyzed 3 hours after the operation and on the next morning respectively.

患者：好的。那鼻胆管我应该注意点什么？

P：All right. What should I pay attention to for the nasobiliary tube?

护士：第一，我们会妥善固定鼻胆管，在鼻孔处我们会用胶布做一个记号，您在洗脸的时候要特别注意，要观察鼻胆管有无脱出，我们会每日更换固定胶布。第二，鼻胆管接负压引流袋，避免打折、扭曲，保证引流通畅，特别是睡觉、翻身时不能压住引流管。第三，注意观察引流液的颜色、性质及量，如果有异常，及时告知医生或护理人员。

N：Firstly, we will properly secure the nasobiliary tube

and mark with a tape on your nostril. You should pay special attention whether the tube slides out or not when washing your face. We will replace the tape every day. Secondly, the nasobiliary tube is connected to a vacuum drainage bag, which should avoid kink, distortion. Make sure it is unobstructed, and do not squeeze the drainage tube when sleeping or turning over. Finally, you must pay attention to the color, nature and volume of the drainage fluid. If something is unusual, please inform the doctor or nursing staff in time.

患者：术后我可以吃东西吗？

P：Can I have foods after the surgery?

护士：术后一般禁饮食 24 小时，或根据病情禁食，遵医嘱补液，防止发生低血糖。第 2 天血淀粉酶正常，无腹痛、恶心、呕吐等症状后，进少量温开水。无异常后，可进流食，以后再半流食，清淡饮食，逐渐过渡为普通低脂饮食。要少量多餐，进低脂、高蛋白、易消化的饮食。

N：After the surgery, patients are generally not allowed to eat or drink for 24 hours, or need to fast according to their condition. We will also give intravenous fluid to prevent hypoglycemia. On the second day, you may drink a little warm water if you have a normal blood amylase level and no symptoms such as abdominal pain, nausea, vomiting are observed. If no abnormal reaction occurs after drinking, you can eat a small amount of liquid foods, then gradually convert to the semi-liquid diet, light diet, and then normal low-fat diet. You should have a low-fat, high-protein and digestible diet in a less and more frequent meals fashion.

患者：好的，谢谢您!

P：OK，thank you!

护士：不用谢!

N：You are welcome!

[Phrases]

inform sb. of	通知某人……
be established on	基于……建立
the basis of	……的基础
duodenal papilla	十二指肠乳头
bile duct	胆管
achieve the aim of	达到……目的
Oddi sphincter	Oddi 括约肌
urine amylase	尿淀粉酶

Specialized Nursing

专科护理

1. Health Education for Patients with Upper Gastrointestinal Hemorrhage
上消化道出血患者的健康教育

[Glossary]

hematemesis	呕血
wipe	擦拭
dizzy	头晕眼花的
pulse	脉搏
prescribe	开处方
hematochezia	便血
consciousness	意识
vomit	呕吐

[Scenario]

家属：护士，护士，快点来，我老公又呕血了。

F：Nurse, come, quick! My husband is vomiting blood.

护士：阿姨，您不要慌张，我来擦擦血渍，现在感觉怎么样？

N：Relax, madam. Let me wipe off the blood. How are you now?

患者：我有点头晕。

P：I'm a little dizzy.

护士：请您先躺下来，头偏向一侧。（呼叫值班医生）医生，23床呕血了，请您抓紧时间过来一下。您不要紧张，我先给您数个脉搏、呼吸。

N：Would you please lie down and turn your head to one side? (call the doctor on call) Doctor, the patient in bed 23 has hematemesis, please come to have a look. Don't be nervous. I'll measure your rates of pulse and breath first.

家属：他怎么样？

F: How is he doing?

护士：脉搏有点快。阿姨，请您拿个盆过来。

N: The pulse is a bit fast. Madam, please bring a basin here.

家属：好的。

F: OK.

医生：现在患者情况怎么样？

D: How is the patient doing now?

护士：患者意识清楚，心率：98 次/分，呼吸：22 次/分，血压：95/43 mmhg。刚刚呕了约 200 ml 鲜血，今天这是第二次了，总量有 500 ml。

N: The patient is conscious. HR：98/min；R：22/min；BP：95/43mmHg. He just vomited about 200 ml of blood. It was the second time today，about 500 ml in total.

医生：给他建立静脉通道了吗？我要给他使用一些止血药。

D: Did you give him a venous access? I'll give him some hemostatic.

护士：建了。

N: Yes，I did.

医生：现在他不能吃东西，需要禁食一段时间。

D: Now he is not allowed to eat and must fast for some time.

护士：好的，我知道了。

N: OK，I see.

患者：我现在感觉好一些了。

P: I feel better now.

医生：给他上个心电监护，血压、脉搏、呼吸、氧饱和度半小时一次，我给他开一些止血药物。

D: Set up an ECG monitor for him, record his blood pressure, pulse, breath, oxygen saturation half an hour, and I'll prescribe some hemostatic medicine.

护士：好的，需不需给他接个氧气？

N：OK, do we need to give him oxygen?

医生：需要，氧流量 5 L/分。

D：Yes, the oxygen flow rate should be 5 L/min.

患者：谢谢你们。

P：Thank you.

医生：请持续监测生命体征变化，并观察有无呕血、便血。

D：Please continuously monitor his vital signs, and observe whether hematemesis or hematochezia happens.

护士：好的。

N：All right.

医生：我现在去开医嘱，有事情及时叫我。

D：I'm going to prescribe the orders now. Please call me if anything happens.

护士：好的。

N：OK.

医生：如果患者还出血就通知血库，做好输血准备，现在给他做个血常规以及血型鉴定。

D：If the patient keeps bleeding, inform the blood bank and prepare for blood transfusion. Now give him a blood test and blood type identification test.

护士：好的，叔叔您现在休息一下，不要起来，我担心您会跌倒。

N：All right. Sir, please have a rest now, and do not get up, as we don't want to see you fall down.

患者：我知道了，谢谢。

P：I see, thank you.

[Phrases]

on call	值班
venous access	静脉通道
ECG monitor	心电监护

oxygen saturation	氧饱和度
oxygen flow	氧流量
continuously monitor	持续监测
vital sign	生命体征
blood transfusion	输血
blood type identification	血型鉴定

2. Health Education for Patients with Ascites
腹水患者的健康教育

[Glossary]

ascites	腹水
edema	水肿
intake and output	出入量
lower limb	下肢
blood coagulation function	凝血功能
intra-abdominal pressure	腹内压

[Scenario]

护士：您好！张先生！我是您的责任护士春梅。

N：Hello! Mr. Zhang! I am the nurse in charge of you. My name is Chunmei.

患者：你好！春梅。

P：Hello! Chunmei.

护士：因为您有腹水，我来给您做个腹水的宣教。

N：Since you have ascites, I'll give you a health education about it.

患者：好的，谢谢你！

P：Good, thank you!

护士：因为您有腹水，双下肢也水肿了，所以您每天喝的水不能太多，应限制在 1 000 ml 左右。您要每天准确记录您的出入量，这样便于观察病情，并为医生用药提供可靠的资料。

N：Because of ascites, and both of your lower limbs are edematous, please do not drink too much water, limit your water intake to the amount of about 1 000 ml a day. Remember to record the intake and output accurately, which is helpful for analyzing your condition and providing the doctor with reliable information for prescribing.

患者：好的，我会认真记的。

P：OK，I'll do it carefully.

护士：肝功能不好的患者，凝血功能也会不好，食管、胃底曲张的静脉很容易出血，所以您不能吃那些硬的、粗糙的食物，要吃柔软的。不要吃太油腻的食物，尽量清淡。平时饮食要少盐或者无盐，不能吃太咸的，如咸菜、酱菜等。此外，要少食多餐，细嚼慢咽。

N：Patients with poor liver function usually have poor blood coagulation function too, and esophageal and gastric varices are easy to bleed, so you should eat soft foods instead of hard and rough foods. In addition, avoid greasy foods, and a light diet is suggested. Diets should contain a little salt or no salt. Salty foods such as pickles and marinated vegetables should be avoided. Eat less and more frequently. And please chew your food carefully before swallowing it.

患者：那我应该吃些什么呢？

P：What should I eat?

护士：要加强营养，您可以适量吃些蛋白质含量高的食物，如牛奶、鸡蛋、瘦肉等，多吃些新鲜的水果、蔬菜。

N：You are suggested to eat high-protein foods, such as milk, eggs and lean meats to improve your nutrition. In addition, you should have more fresh fruits and vegetables.

患者：我知道了。那平时要注意些什么吗？

P：I see. What should I pay attention to?

护士：可以经常抬高双下肢，减轻水肿。尽量避免用力咳嗽和用力排便，以免加重腹内压，加重腹胀，造成不舒服。

N：You can frequently raise the lower limbs to reduce edema. Try to avoid hard cough and forced defecation，so as not to increase the intra-abdominal pressure，which may aggravate abdominal distension and discomfort.

患者：好的！那我能活动吗？

P：OK！Can I do some exercises?

护士：可以的，您可以适当活动，多注意休息，不要太劳累，如果感到不舒服就停下来。尽量保持心情愉悦，好的心态对恢复疾病很有用。同时，还要注意个人卫生，注意保暖，不要感冒了！

N：Yes，you can take part in some moderate activities，have good rests，limit the intensity and stop doing any activities whenever you feel uncomfortable. Try to keep a good mood，which will be very beneficial to your recovery. Meanwhile，pay attention to your personal hygiene and keep warm for avoiding catching a cold!

患者：好的，谢谢你！

P：OK，thank you!

护士：不用谢！祝您早日康复！

N：My pleasure! Wish you recover soon!

[Phrases]

catch a cold	感冒
keep warm	保暖
be very beneficial to	非常有益于
poor liver function	肝功能不好
in charge of	负责

3. Health Education for Patients with Portal Hypertension
门静脉高压症患者的健康教育

[Glossary]

portal	门静脉
hypertension	高压
circulation	循环
splenomegaly	脾大
ascites	腹水
characteristic	特有的
optimistic	乐观的
regeneration	再生
glucose	葡萄糖
hematemesis	呕血
melena	黑便

[Scenario]

患者：李护士，医生今天给我说，我们门静脉高压，我没太听明白，你能给我再解释解释吗？

P: Nurse Li, the doctor said that I have portal hypertension. I did not quite understand. Would you please explain it to me?

护士：钱先生，门静脉高压是因为各种原因引起了门静脉系统血流阻力增大，血流量增加超过了门静脉循环的顺应性导致的。它主要表现在：脾脏肿大、腹水、门体侧支循环的形成及门脉高压性胃肠病，其中以门体侧支循环的形成最具特征性。

N: Mr. Qian, portal hypertension is caused by the increase of portal venous blood flow resistance due to a variety of reasons. When increased blood flow exceeds the portal vein circulation capacity, it may lead to portal hypertension. The main symptoms include: splenomegaly, ascites, formation of portosystemic collateral circulation and portal hypertensive gastrointestinal disease, among which the formation of portosystemic collateral circulation is the most characteristic.

患者：我自己能做些什么？

P：What shall I do?

护士：您要保持心情乐观，避免情绪紧张。休息有利于肝脏微循环的改善，促进肝细胞再生修复，减轻肝损害。您的情况还不严重，可适当参加一些活动，但减少劳动时间及劳动强度。注意劳逸结合，保证足够的卧床休息及睡眠时间。

N：You need to keep an optimistic mood and avoid emotional stress. Resting can improve liver microcirculation. It can also promote the regeneration and repair of liver cells, and reduce liver damage. Your situation is not serious. You may participate in some moderate activities. But you should keep an eye on the time and intensity. You need to alternate work with rest and ensure adequate bed rest and sleeping time.

患者：我会的。

P：I will.

护士：您可以多吃富含维生素的食物，食物中除含有高糖、高蛋白质、适当脂肪外，还应含有各种无机盐及微量元素。食物以高糖为主，如米、面、谷类。蛋白质每天给予 100 g 左右，尽量选用富含各种氨基酸的蛋白质，如鱼、瘦肉、禽、蛋、奶及豆制品等。脂肪一般不宜过多，每天 30～50 g 即可。尽量不要吃辛辣刺激性食物，严禁饮酒。

N：You can eat foods with rich vitamin，high glucose，high protein and appropriate fat. Meanwhile，foods should also contain all kinds of inorganic salts and microelements. You'd better mainly take foods with high sugar such as rice，flour and cereals. The protein intake should be around 100 g every day，and try to choose the protein rich in different types of amino acids，such as fish，lean meat，poultry，eggs，milk，soy bean products，and so on. Do not eat too much fat，no more than 30~50 g per day. You should avoid spicy and pungent foods. Alcohol is strictly prohibited.

患者：那我回家要注意什么？

P：What should I pay attention to when I go back home？

护士：您还需要按医嘱用护肝、降酶、退黄药物治疗。出院后每 2~3 个月随访一次，复查血常规、肝功能、甲胎蛋白等，注意有无黄疸、腹水、呕血和黑便。

N：You also need to take medications for liver protection，enzyme reduction，and jaundice treatment according to the doctor's advice. Do not forget to come back for follow-ups every 2 ~ 3 months after discharge to recheck your blood count，liver function，alpha fetoprotein（AFP），and observe if there are jaundice，ascites，hematemesis and melena.

患者：谢谢，我能要一下你们的电话吗？我想有问题时再咨询你们。

P：Thank you. May I have your phone number？I'd like to ask you again if I have any questions.

护士：好的，我给您写在纸上。

N：OK，I will write it on the paper.

[Phrases]

be caused by	由……引起
a variety of	各种
blood flow	血流
collateral circulation	侧支循环
gastrointestinal disease	胃肠道疾病
emotional stress	情绪紧张
microcirculation	微循环
participate in	参加
inorganic salt	无机盐
microelement	微量元素
amino acid	氨基酸
alpha fetoprotein（AFP）	甲胎蛋白

4. Health Education for Patients with Hepatic Hemangioma
肝血管瘤患者的健康教育

[Glossary]

hepatic	肝的
hemangioma	血管瘤
interventional	介入的
therapy	治疗
puncture	穿刺
angiography	血管造影
embolization	栓塞

[Scenario]

护士：您好,1 床阿姨,请问您叫什么名字?

N：Hello! Madam. What's your name?

患者：护士你好,我叫李莉。

P：Hello. My name is Li Li.

护士：李阿姨,医生已经给您制订了手术方案,肝血管瘤介入治疗!

N：Ms. Li, the doctor has decided the treatment for you. The hepatic hemangioma interventional therapy!

患者：太好了,谢谢。那我要做些什么准备?

P：That's great, thank you. So what should I do?

护士：介入手术是微创手术,请您不要担心! 术前 4 小时禁食、禁水。您可以先去洗个澡,更换清洁衣裤。

N：Interventional operation is a minimally invasive surgery. Please don't worry! Don't eat or drink 4 hours before the operation. You can take a shower first and put on some clean clothes.

患者：好的！

P: OK!

护士：我们一般经股动脉穿刺插管，选择或超选择造影，明确肝血管瘤的大小、部位、数目。然后将导管头端超选至血管瘤的供血动脉进行缓慢栓塞。栓塞完毕行肝动脉造影以评定栓塞效果。最后拔出导管用加压器进行加压止血就可以了！

N: This operation is usually done by puncture and catheterization from the femoral artery. The size, location and number of lesions of the hepatic hemangioma will be confirmed by selective or superselective angiography. The tip of the catheter will be sent to the feeding artery of the hemangioma, which is then embolized slowly. Hepatic arteriography will be performed after the embolization to evaluate the effect of the treatment. Finally, pull out the catheter and apply pressure to the puncture site with a tourniquet to prevent bleeding!

患者：谢谢，那我手术回来要注意一些什么吗？

P: Thank you. What should I pay attention to after the operation?

护士：术后 2 小时内禁食、水，8 小时保持术肢制动，12 小时才能下床活动。术后可能会有腹痛、恶心、呕吐、发热等情况！请不要担心，这都是术后正常反应，您只需要告知我们，我们会给您对症处理的！

N: Don't eat or drink within 2 hours after the surgery, and keep the operated limb immobilized within 8 hours. You can get out of the bed 12 hours after the surgery. Abdominal pain, nausea, vomiting, fever may occur, but don't worry. These symptoms are normal postoperative reactions. You just need to tell us and we'll give you appropriate treatments!

患者：知道了！

P: I see!

护士：术后多食高热量、高蛋白质、高维生素、低脂肪食物，多食水果、蔬菜。保持大便通畅，避免用力排便，以免增加腹腔压力，引起瘤体破裂出血。希望对您有所帮助。

N: After the surgery, you need diets with high calorie, high protein, high vitamin and low fat, and eat more fruits and vegetables. Keep your bowels move, and don't defecate forcefully to avoid a sudden increase in abdominal pressure as it may cause rupture and bleeding of the lesion. I hope this is helpful to you.

患者：帮助非常大，谢谢，我现在没有那么紧张了，那我回家要注意什么呢？

P: It is very helpful. Thank you. I am not so nervous now, then what should I pay attention to when I go back home?

护士：回家要保持心情舒畅，避免激烈的情绪变化，积极参加文娱活动，保持生活规律。忌剧烈运动及重体力劳动，避免外力碰撞，定期随访。

N: You should keep a good mood at home, avoid sudden and strong emotional changes, take an active part in recreational activities, and keep a regular life style. Avoid strenuous exercises and heavy physical labor, avoid external collision, and do not forget the regular follow-ups with us.

患者：好的，谢谢。

P: OK, thank you.

护士：不客气，有需要再找我。

N: You're welcome. Please let me know if you need any help.

[**Phrases**]

interventional operation	介入手术
minimally invasive surgery	微创手术
femoral artery	股动脉
abdominal pain	腹痛
high calorie	高热量
abdominal pressure	腹压
regular life style	规律生活

5. Health Education for Pain Patients
   疼痛患者的健康教育

[Glossary]

continuous	持续的
intermittent	间断的
analgesic	止疼剂
tumor	肿瘤
indomethacin	吲哚美辛
suppository	栓剂
aspirin	阿司匹林
moderate	中等的
tramadol	曲马多
morphine	吗啡
dizziness	眩晕
constipation	便秘

[Scenario]

护士：您好！我是您的责任护士春梅。
N：Hi! I'm your primary nurse Chunmei.

患者：你好！
P：Hi!

护士：请问您现在有哪里不舒服吗？
N：How are you feeling today?

患者：我肚子痛。
P：I have an abdominal pain.

护士：是哪个部位痛啊？您用手指给我看看，好吗？
N：Where exactly is the pain? Would you please point it
   out with your finger?

患者：这里。
P：Here.

护士：您痛了多长时间啦？

N：How long have you been like this?

患者：2个月了。

P：2 months.

护士：痛是持续的还是间歇的呢？

N：Is the pain continuous or intermittent?

患者：持续的，我一直在吃这个药（泰勒宁）。

P：It's continuous，and I have been taking this medicine （tylox）.

护士：这是我们评估疼痛的痛尺，从1到10分，您觉得您现在的疼痛有几分？

N：This is the scale we use for pain assessment，from 1 to 10，what score do you think the pain is?

患者：2分，我半小时前刚吃了止痛药，现在好点了。

P：2，I just took an analgesic half an hour ago，now I feel better.

护士：吃这个药能控制您的疼痛吗？

N：Can this medicine control your pain?

患者：以前可以的，最近吃这个药之后2小时就会再次疼痛。

P：It could，but now the pain comes back 2 hours after taking this medicine.

护士：现在这个药不能很好地控制您的疼痛，得换种止痛药了。对于肿瘤引起的慢性疼痛，一般我们会选择三阶梯止痛。

N：As this medicine can no longer control you pain well，we suggest you to change. For the chronic pain caused by tumor，we usually choose the three-step ladder cancer pain management.

患者：什么是三阶梯止痛？

P：What is three-step ladder cancer pain management?

护士：根据疼痛的程度分别选择不同阶梯的止痛药物。轻度疼痛选择非阿片类药物，如吲哚美辛栓，阿司匹林等。中度疼痛选择弱阿片类药物,如曲马多,泰勒宁等。重度疼痛选择强阿片类药物,如吗啡,芬太尼贴剂等。现在可能吗啡类的止痛药才能更好地控制您的疼痛了。

N：According to the degree of the pain，we choose different analgesic drugs for different intensity. Non-opioid drugs are used for mild pain，such as indomethacin suppositories，aspirin and others. Mild opioid drugs are used for moderate pain，such as tramadol，tylox and others. Strong opioid drugs are used for severe pain，such as morphine，fentanyl patches and others. You may now have to choose morphine-based painkillers to control your pain.

患者：吗啡类的止痛药吃了会成瘾吗? 有什么副作用吗?

P：Are morphine-based painkillers addictive? Are there any side effects?

护士：不会成瘾。吃了吗啡类的止痛药可能会出现头晕、恶心、呕吐、便秘等不良反应,但不是每个人都会有症状。

N：There won't be addiction. They do have some side effects such as dizziness，nausea，vomiting and constipation. However，the severity varies among the patients.

患者：好的,我知道了! 谢谢你!

P：OK，I got it. Thank you very much!

护士：不客气! 我会将您的情况告诉医生。

N：You're welcome! I will tell your doctor about your situation.

患者：谢谢你。

P：Thank you.

护士：不用谢。

N：My pleasure.

[Phrases]

abdominal pain	腹痛
pain assessment	疼痛评估
chronic pain	慢性疼痛
three-step ladder	三阶梯
pain management	疼痛管理
mild pain	轻度疼痛
non-opioid drug	非阿片类药物
mild opioid drug	弱阿片类药物
strong opioid drug	强阿片类药物
severe pain	重度疼痛
fentanyl patch	芬太尼贴剂

6. Health Education for Fever Patients
发热患者的健康教育

[Glossary]

fever	发热
thermometer	体温表
take the temperature	量体温
ice compress	冰敷
alcohol bath	酒精擦浴

[Scenario]

护士：李先生，您好！我是您的责任护士孙芋，您现在有哪里不舒服吗？

N：Hello! Mr. Li! I am the nurse in charge of you, and my name is Sun Qian. How do you feel now?

患者：小孙，您好！我现在好像有点发热。

P：Hello, Xiao Sun! It seems I have a fever.

护士：好的，那我去拿体温表给您测量一下体温。

N：OK, I'll get the thermometer to take your temperature.

患者：好的。

P：All right.

护士：李先生，请把这个体温表夹到腋下 5 分钟，我等一会过来看。

N：Mr. Li, please put the thermometer under your armpit for 5 minutes. I'll check you up a moment later.

患者：嗯，知道了。

P：Oh, I will.

护士：您现在的体温是 37.5 ℃，稍微有点低烧。

N：Your temperature is 37.5 ℃. You have a mild fever.

患者：很严重吗？

P：Is it serious?

护士：由于术后大量肿瘤组织坏死及正常细胞受损，患者
　　　均可出现体温升高，一般在 38.5 ℃左右，无需特殊
　　　处理，3～5 天自然缓解。

N：The rise of body temperature is caused by tumor
　　necrosis and the damage of normal liver cells after the
　　treatment. The temperature is usually around 38.5 ℃.
　　No special treatment is needed as it can be naturally
　　relieved within 3 to 5 days.

患者：可是我感觉比之前更热了。

P：But I feel even hotter than before now.

护士：您不要担心，如果高热不退，我们会给予冰敷、酒精
　　　擦浴等方式给您降温，或者服用一些药物，您很快就
　　　会好起来的。

N：Don't worry. We will give you some ice compression or
　　alcohol bath to reduce your body temperature if the
　　high fever persists. We will also give you some
　　medicines if necessary. You will get better soon.

患者：那我现在需要做点什么吗？

P：What should I do then?

护士：您现在要多饮水，除了有点低热，还有其他的不
　　　适吗？

N：Please drink more water. Do you feel any other
　　discomfort except the fever?

患者：好的，没有了。

P：No.

护士：那 30 分钟以后再复测一下体温，如果有什么不舒服
　　　请及时按铃，呼叫铃在床旁边，我也会经常来看
　　　您的。

N：Please recheck the temperature 30 minutes later. If
　　you feel uncomfortable，please ring the bell in time.
　　The bell is at the bedside. Also，I will come to see you
　　regularly.

患者：好的，谢谢你。
P：OK，thank you.
护士：不客气。
N：It's my pleasure.

[Phrases]

recheck the temperature	复测体温
ring the bell	按铃
reduce the fever	降温

7. Health Education for Patients with Allergic Reactions
发生过敏反应患者的健康教育

[Glossary]

stool	大便
urine	小便
itchy	瘙痒的
dyspnea	呼吸困难
chemotherapy	化疗
oxaliplatin	奥沙利铂
allergy	过敏

[Scenario]

护士：徐兵，昨晚睡得好吗？

N：Xu Bing, did you sleep well last night?

患者：还可以，睡了 5 小时。

P：Not bad, I slept for 5 hours.

护士：吃早饭了吗？

N：Did you have breakfast?

患者：吃了，吃了半碗稀饭，一个包子。

P：Yes, I had half a bowl of porridge and a bun.

护士：很好！昨天大小便怎么样？

N：Very good! What about the stool and urine yesterday?

患者：大小便都正常！

P：Both were fine.

护士：小便什么颜色？

N：What was the color of the urine?

患者：昨天手术后，你不是让我多饮水吗？我喝了很多水，我的小便是淡黄色的。

P：According to your instruction, I drank a lot of water

after the surgery yesterday, and my urine was pale yellow.

护士：那很好，我怎么觉得你的脸有点红，你现在有什么不舒服吗？

N：Great. I think your face is a little red. Any discomfort?

患者：早上起来后身上就有点痒。

P：I felt a little itchy after I got up in the morning.

护士：那让我看看（拉窗帘），什么时候开始的？

N：Let me see（draw the curtains），When did this symptom start?

患者：早上起来就有点痒了，现在痒得更厉害了，昨天还好好的。

P：Yesterday it was fine，but I felt a little itchy after getting up in the morning，and now it is getting worse.

护士：你可能对昨天手术过程中使用的某个药物过敏。

N：You may be allergic to some medicine used in the operation yesterday.

护士：呼吸怎么样？觉得呼吸困难吗？

N：How is your breathing? Do you have dyspnea?

患者：呼吸没什么问题，除了痒，没有其他不舒服了。

P：My breathing is OK. Apart from the itchiness, there's no other discomfort.

护士：你不要用手抓挠皮肤，不要用肥皂洗澡，穿宽松一点的棉质衣物。我会告知医生，让他过来看你。

N：Don't scratch the skin，or use soap for bathing，wear loose cotton clothes. I'll ask the doctor to check on you.

患者：好的，谢谢你，你说我有可能对什么过敏？

P：All right，thank you. What do you think may I be allergic to?

护士：手术中你使用的化疗药物是奥沙利铂，但治疗过程中你也用了对比剂，也会导致过敏。你的这种情况很像对比剂的变态反应中的皮肤反应,是过敏反应中较轻的一种。

N：The chemotherapy drug you used during the surgery is oxaliplatin, but during the treatment you also used a contrast agent, which can lead to allergies as well. Your situation is a bit like the skin reaction of contrast agent allergy, which is a slight one though.

患者：我知道了,谢谢。

P：I got it. Thank you.

护士：没事,我现在去叫医生,如果你有哪里不舒服,就按铃。

N：You're welcome. I am going to inform the doctor of your situation. Just ring the bell if you need me.

[Phrases]

a bowl of	一碗
pale yellow	淡黄色
be allergic to	对……过敏
loose cotton clothes	宽松棉质衣物
contrast agent	对比剂
lead to	导致
skin reaction	皮肤反应

8. Health Education for Patients with Hematoma
血肿患者的健康教育

[Glossary]

hematoma	血肿
bloated	肿胀的
defecate	排便
forcibly	用力地
absorption	吸收
emphasis	强调
enlargement	扩大
rehabilitation	康复
unfavorable	不利的
extubation	拔管

[Scenario]

护士：李阿姨，您好，今天是您介入手术后的第二天，您现在感觉怎么样？

N：Hello，Ms. Li. Today is the second day after your interventional operation. How do you feel now?

患者：没有什么特殊的感觉，就是昨天手术的地方有点胀，有点疼。

P：Nothing special. I just feel a little bit bloated and painful in the operation site.

护士：可以让我看一下手术的地方吗？

N：Can I take a look?

患者：好的。

P：Of course.

护士：您的手术穿刺点有点肿，可能是发生了血肿。

N：Your puncture point is swollen and there may be a

hematoma.

患者：什么是血肿？我不太明白。很严重吗？怎么会这样啊？

P：What is hematoma? I do not understand. Is it serious? Why did it happen?

护士：阿姨,您不要这么紧张,股动脉穿刺术后是有可能发生血肿的,还好我们发现得早,采取一些简单的措施就可以让血肿慢慢吸收消失了。

N：Ms. Li, take it easy. It is possible to have the hematoma after the femoral artery puncture. Fortunately, we found it early and it will disappear by some simple measures. The hematoma will be absorbed gradually.

患者：要用什么办法啊？

P：What is the measure?

护士：因为您现在出现了血肿,所以需要延长加压包扎的时间。您在咳嗽或者用力排便、排尿时要压迫穿刺点。如果您的穿刺点出血的话,我们会给您重新加压包扎。出现血肿 24 小时后,我们可以热敷伤口以促进吸收。现在的重点还是加压包扎以及防止血肿继续扩大。

N：Because you have a hematoma now, you need to use pressure bandage a bit longer. You should press the puncture point when you cough, defecate forcibly or urinate. If your puncture point bleeds, we will reapply the pressure bandage for you. After 24 hours of hematoma, we can use warm compress for the wound to promote absorption. The emphasis now is on pressure bandage and prevention of continued enlargement of the hematoma.

患者：那我可以活动吗？我躺在床上时间太久了,很难受。

P：Can I move around? I've been lying in bed for too long. I feel so uncomfortable.

护士：阿姨，我理解您的感受，任何人躺在床上时间长了都不会舒服的，但是您现在的情况不适合下床活动。您需要卧床休息，防止伤口继续出血，那样的话血肿会持续扩大，不利于康复。希望您能理解并配合我们的工作，这都是为了您好。

N：Ms. Li, I know your feelings. Anyone lying in bed for such a long time would not feel well. However, your situation is not suitable for getting out of bed. You have to rest in bed to prevent the wound from further bleeding. If the bleeding continues and hematoma enlarges, it will be unfavorable for your rehabilitation. I hope you can understand and cooperate with us. It is all for your own good.

患者：好的，我明白了。那为什么我会出现血肿？我想了解一下。

P：OK，I see. What is the cause of hematoma? I want to know about it.

护士：血肿产生的原因很多，主要有：反复穿刺插管、拔管后穿刺点压迫不当、肝素用量过大或患者自身存在凝血功能障碍。

N：There are many reasons to cause a hematoma. It is mainly due to repeated puncture, improper compression after extubation, overdose of heparin, or coagulation disorders of patients.

患者：那我是哪种原因引起的呢？

P：Which one caused mine?

护士：这个我现在还不能确定，需要医生对您做身体评估以及相关检查之后才能确定。我一会儿会把您的情况告知您的管床医生的，您不要太担心。

N：I'm not sure yet. You need the doctor to make a physical assessment and related examinations. I'll tell your doctor about it later. Don't worry too much.

患者：好的，太感谢您了。

P：OK, thank you very much.

护士：不用客气，这是我应该做的，您好好休息。

N：Don't mention it. That's what I should do. Have a good rest.

患者：好的，谢谢。

P：OK, thank you.

[Phrases]

femoral artery	股动脉
pressure bandage	加压包扎
cooperate with	合作
repeated puncture	反复穿刺
improper compression	压迫不当
coagulation disorder	凝血功能障碍

9. Health Education for Patients with Hypokalemia After Transcatheter Arterial Chemoembolization
肝癌栓塞术后低钾血症患者的健康教育

[Glossary]

hypokalemia	低钾血症
transcatheter	经导管
chemoembolization	化疗栓塞
supplement	补充

[Scenario]

护士：李先生，早上好。我是您的责任护士春梅。

N：Mr. Li, good morning. I am your primary nurse Chunmei.

患者：早上好。

P：Good morning.

护士：您昨天做了肝栓塞化疗，今天感觉怎么样？有什么不舒服的吗？

N：You had transcatheter arterial chemoembolization (TACE) yesterday, how are you feeling today? Is there any discomfort?

患者：没有什么特别的感觉，就是浑身无力，不想动，不想吃东西。

P：Nothing special, I just feel weak, and do not want to move or eat.

护士：您今天早上抽血检查了吗？

N：Did you take the blood test this morning?

患者：是的，5 点多的时候值班护士过来给我抽血，她说结果会在早上 8 点多出来。

P：Yes, at 5 o'clock, the nurse on call came to draw blood for me. She said the blood test result would come out at

8 in the morning.

护士：好的，我一会儿去护士站的电脑给您看一下血液检
　　　查的结果。

N：OK，I'll go to the nurse station and check your result
　　on the computer later.

患者：好的，谢谢你。

P：All right，thank you.

护士：李先生，您的血液检查结果已经出来了，其他血液指
　　　标都还可以，但是血钾有点低，是 2.9 mmol/L。

N：Mr. Li，your blood test result has come out. It seems
　　fine except that the blood potassium is a bit low. It is
　　2.9 mmol/L.

患者：很低吗？正常值是多少呢？

P：Is it very low？ What is the normal value？

护士：这个值低于正常血钾值，但不是特别低。正常血钾
　　　范围是 3.5～5.5 mmol/L。

N：It is lower than normal，but not particularly low. The
　　range of normal blood potassium is 3.5～5.5 mmol/L.

患者：哦，那我现在要怎么办？

P：Oh，what am I going to do now？

护士：您不要紧张，低钾血症是肝癌栓塞化疗术后经常发
　　　生的症状。您现在的血钾没有特别低，并不是非常
　　　严重。您可以少量多餐，尽量多吃点高钾食物。

N：You don't have to be nervous. Hypokalemia is
　　common after TACE. Your blood potassium is not
　　very low，so it is not a serious condition. You can eat
　　less and more often and try to eat foods rich in
　　potassium.

患者：哪些是高钾食物呢？我不太清楚。

P：What are the foods with rich potassium？ I have no
　　idea.

护士：高钾的食物有很多种。水果里面有：香蕉、苹果、葡

萄、西瓜、杏子、橘子;蔬菜里面有:菠菜、苋菜、香菜、油菜、甘蓝、茄子、番茄、黄瓜、芹菜等;海藻类里面有:紫菜、海带等。您可以根据自己的喜好,选择一些喜欢吃的食物,定时定量,多吃一点。

N: There are many kinds of high-potassium foods. For fruits we have banana, apple, grape, watermelon, apricot, orange, etc.; for vegetables we have spinach, amaranth, coriander, rape, cabbage, eggplant, tomato, cucumber, celery, etc.; for seaweed foods we have nori, kelp, etc. You may choose those you preferred, and take a certain amount of them regularly.

患者:好的,我明白了。那要是吃这些食物不管用怎么办?低钾血症会不会恶化?

P: All right, I see. What can I do if it does not work after I eat these foods? Will the hypokalemia get worse?

护士:这些食物会有帮助的,您不要太担心。如果您通过饮食疗法不能改善低钾血症或者您的情况继续恶化,医生会给您开一些口服补钾的药物,因为口服补钾效果好,而且更安全。有极少部分患者会出现严重低血钾的情况,我们会采用静脉补钾的方法。

N: These foods will be helpful. Don't worry too much. If your hypokalemia is not improved by diet therapy, or your condition keeps getting worse, the doctor will give you some oral potassium supplement because oral potassium supplement is better and safer. For those rare severe hypokalemia patients, we will supplement potassium intravenously.

患者:好的,我明白了。

P: OK, I see.

护士:那您让您家里人先去买一些香蕉、苹果之类的高钾水果吧,等到中午吃饭的时候再买一些其他的高钾食物。

N: You can ask your family to buy some high-potassium fruits such as bananas and apples, and buy some other high-potassium foods at lunch time.

患者：好。

P: OK.

护士：那您好好休息，有什么问题请您随时告诉我。

N: Have a good rest. Please let me know if you have any questions.

患者：好的，谢谢。

P: All right, thank you.

护士：不用客气。

N: You are welcome.

[Phrases]

blood test	血液检查
come out	出来
nurse station	护士站
blood potassium	血钾
normal value	正常值
particularly low	特别低
diet therapy	饮食疗法
oral potassium supplement	口服补钾

10. Health Education for Diabetic Patients
　　糖尿病患者的健康教育

［Glossary］

diabetes	糖尿病
insulin	胰岛素
hereditary	遗传的
metabolic	代谢的
hyperglycemia	高血糖
deficiency	缺陷
dysfunction	功能障碍
obesity	肥胖

［Scenario］

护士：张阿姨，您好。
N：Hello，Ms. Zhang.

患者：小李，你好。
P：Hello，Xiao li.

护士：您昨晚睡得怎么样？
N：How was your sleep last night?

患者：我昨晚睡得很好。
P：Very well.

护士：您几点钟吃早饭？
N：When will you have breakfast?

患者：现在还不确定，可能再过半个小时吧，我老公去给我
　　　买早饭了。
P：I'm not sure yet，maybe half an hour later. My
　　husband went out to buy me breakfast.

护士：好的，您吃早饭之前不要忘记打胰岛素。
N：All right. Don't forget to inject insulin before
　　breakfast.

患者：不会忘记的，我每天都记得，早饭前半个小时打 4 个
　　　单位。

P：I won't. I do it every day-inject 4 units half an hour
　　before breakfast.

护士：非常好，您得糖尿病多久了？

N：Very good. How long have you had diabetes?

患者：大概 20 年了，具体我也记不太清楚。我的血糖一直
　　　控制得很好，但是我对糖尿病的认识并不多。你能
　　　给我讲讲吗？

P：About 20 years. I don't remember the exact date. My
　　blood sugar has been under control，but my knowledge
　　of diabetes is little. Can you tell me something about
　　it?

护士：当然可以，那我今天就给您讲讲糖尿病的病因和平
　　　时需要注意的事项，好吗？

N：Of course, I'll tell you about the cause of diabetes and
　　what to pay attention to, OK?

患者：好的。

P：OK.

护士：糖尿病是一组以高血糖为特征的代谢性疾病。高血
　　　糖则是由胰岛素分泌缺陷或其生物作用受损，或两
　　　者兼有引起的。糖尿病时长期存在的高血糖，导致
　　　各种组织，特别是眼、肾、心脏、血管、神经的慢性损
　　　害、功能障碍。糖尿病的病因主要有两个：第一个是
　　　遗传因素，1 型和 2 型糖尿病均存在明显的遗传异质
　　　性。糖尿病存在家族发病倾向，1/4～1/2 的患者有
　　　糖尿病家族史。临床上至少有 60 种以上的遗传综
　　　合征可伴有糖尿病。第二个是环境因素，进食过多，
　　　体力活动减少导致的肥胖是 2 型糖尿病最主要的环
　　　境因素，使具有 2 型糖尿病遗传易感性的个体容易
　　　发病。

N：Diabetes mellitus is a collection of metabolic diseases

characterized by hyperglycemia. Hyperglycemia is caused by the deficiency of insulin secretion or the damage of its biological function, or both. Long-term hyperglycemia in diabetes can lead to chronic damage and dysfunction of various tissues, especially of the eyes, kidneys, heart, blood vessels and nerves. There are two main causes of diabetes mellitus: the first is genetic factor, both type 1 and type 2 diabetes mellitus have obvious genetic heterogeneity. They have a tendency of running in a family, $1/4 \sim 1/2$ patients have a family history. Clinically, there are at least 60 genetic syndromes associated with diabetes mellitus. The second is environmental factor, obesity caused by excessive eating and limited physical activity is the most important environmental factor of type 2 diabetes, which makes individuals with genetic susceptibility of type 2 more prone to disease onset.

患者：我可能是遗传的糖尿病，因为我家里有糖尿病的人很多。那得了糖尿病需要注意哪些方面呢？我经常听人说"五驾马车"，那是什么意思？

P: My diabetes might be hereditary, because it runs in my family. What should patients pay attention to? I often hear people say "five carriages", what does that mean?

护士：糖尿病是慢性病。如果患者平时能保持健康的生活习惯，正确注射胰岛素、及时服药的话，血糖是可以控制得很好的，也很少会出现严重的并发症。我们经常说的"五架马车"其实是控制血糖的综合方式，包括：饮食控制、运动疗法、药物治疗、血糖监测和糖尿病教育。

N: Diabetes is a chronic disease. If patients keep healthy habits, use insulin and oral medication correctly, the blood glucose can be controlled very well, and serious complications rarely occur. The "five carriages" that we often talk about is actually an integrated way of controlling blood sugar, including diet control, exercise therapy, medication, blood sugar monitoring and diabetes education.

患者：原来如此，今天我终于明白了，你讲得真的非常详细，谢谢！

P: So that is what it is. I finally have a clue today! You really explained in great detail, thank you!

护士：不用谢！您如果还有什么需要了解的，请告诉我，我会及时为您解答的。

N: You are welcome! If you need to know more, please tell me, I will answer you in time.

患者：好的，我觉得这个时间我该注射胰岛素了。

P: That's very nice! Well, I think it's time for me to inject insulin.

护士：好的。

N: OK.

[Phrases]

blood sugar	血糖
be characterized by	以……为特征
insulin secretion	胰岛素分泌
biological function	生物功能
exercise therapy	运动疗法
blood sugar monitoring	血糖监测

11. Health Education for Jaundiced Patients
黄疸患者的健康教育

[Glossary]

jaundice	黄疸
urine	小便
bilirubin	胆红素
high-quality protein	优质蛋白
bile salt	胆盐
clinical manifestation	临床表现

[Scenario]

护士：您好，李先生，我是您的责任护士娴芝。我现在来给您做一下问诊及一些针对性的健康教育。

N：Hello, Mr. Li, I am your primary nurse. My name is Xian Zhi. I am going to ask you some questions and give you some specific health education now.

患者：好的。

P：Great.

护士：请问您是什么时候发现皮肤和巩膜发黄的？

N：When did you notice your skin and sclera turn yellow?

患者：上个月中旬。

P：In the middle of last month.

护士：有一些其他的不正常表现吗？譬如大小便的颜色、身上有无瘙痒等。

N：Are there any other abnormal symptoms? For example, the color of feces and urine, or skin itchiness.

患者：让我想想。好像是的。大便发白，小便发黄。身上在安静时痒得比较厉害。

P：Let me see. Yes. The feces looks white and the urine is

dark yellow. My body itches especially when I'm resting.

护士：好的，这些都是黄疸的一些临床表现。黄疸就是血液中的胆红素过高。出现梗阻性黄疸时，胆汁无法进入肠腔代谢，大便颜色便呈陶土色，而过多的胆红素只能通过泌尿系统代谢，小便颜色就会呈酱油色。胆盐在皮肤下，皮肤就容易瘙痒。

N：OK. These are the clinical manifestations of jaundice. Jaundice is caused by high level of bilirubin in the blood. When obstructive jaundice occurs, the bile may not reach intestinal tract and be metabolized, which makes the color of the feces argil. So the excessive bilirubin can only be excreted through the urinary system, which makes the color of the urine soy sauce. The skin will be itching if the bile salts accumulate under the skin.

患者：那我日常生活中有哪些需要注意的吗？

P：Is there anything I need to pay attention to in my daily life?

护士：首先饮食方面，您不要吃过硬的，如坚果类，应该吃一些优质蛋白、高糖类、高维生素、易消化食物，加强营养。最好不要吃肥肉、油煎、油炸的高脂类食物，不喝浓茶、咖啡。

N：Firstly, you should pay attention to your diets. Don't eat hard foods such as nuts. You should eat digestible foods with rich high-quality protein, carbohydrates and vitamin to strengthen your nutrition. You'd better not eat high-fat foods such as animal fat and fried foods. Strong tea and coffee should also be avoided.

患者：请问什么叫优质蛋白？

P：What is high-quality protein?

护士：一般，动物蛋白都是优质蛋白，植物蛋白里大豆蛋白也是优质蛋白。

N：Animal proteins are generally of high quality. Among the vegetable protein，soybean protein is also of high quality.

患者：其他方面呢？

P：Anything else?

护士：您应该多注意休息。最好晚上 10 点前睡觉，保证 8 小时以上的睡觉时间。平时生活中不可过度劳累，适当活动。

N：You are suggested to take more rest，and go to bed before 10 p.m. Make sure you can sleep for at least 8 hours. Try not to overtire yourself in daily life，and take moderate exercises.

患者：好的。

P：OK.

护士：皮肤瘙痒的时候，自己不要抓挠，避免抓破感染。尽量穿宽松的棉质衣服。实在太痒，可以根据情况让医生给您开点止痒的药膏涂抹。洗澡时，尽量清水洗，避免使用碱性较大的沐浴液、肥皂等。

N：Please don't scratch when you feel itchy to avoid skin infection. Try to wear loose cotton clothes. If the skin is too itching，you can ask the doctor to prescribe some medicines to relieve. Please bath with clean water，do not use alkaline shower gel，soap，etc.

患者：这样啊。

P：I see.

护士：最后，医生会根据您的情况开一些静脉药物来缓解疾病。所以不要太担心，放松心情。

N：Finally，the doctor will prescribe some intravenous medicines to relieve the disease according to your situation. So don't worry too much，be relaxed.

患者：我明白了，凌护士。谢谢你的宣教。

P：I see，Nurse Ling. Thank you for your information.

护士：不客气，应该的。如果有什么其他想知道的，可以来问我。

N：You're welcome. Feel free to reach out to me for any further questions you may have.

患者：谢谢！

P：Thank you！

护士：不用谢。那您注意休息。

N：It is my pleasure. Have a good rest.

[Phrases]

health education	健康教育
urinary system	泌尿系统
in one's daily life	在……的日常生活中

**Health Education for
Hospitalized Patients**

住院患者的健康教育

1. Health Education for Hospital Admission 入院宣教

[Glossary]

drug allergy	药物过敏
hospitalization certificate	住院证
contact number	联系电话
educational background	学历
penicillin	青霉素
diabetes	糖尿病
hypertension	高血压
appetite	食欲
nurse station	护士站

[Scenario]

护士：先生，早上好，您是过来住院的吗？

N：Good morning, sir. Are you here for admission?

患者：是的。

P：Yes.

护士：请把您的住院证给我。

N：May I have your hospitalization certificate please?

患者：好的。

P：Sure. Here it is.

护士：张先生，您好，请问您是第一次住院吗？

N：Is this your first admission, Mr. Zhang?

患者：是的。

P：Yes.

护士：好的，我们这里是介入科，我叫小娜，您可以叫我小李，现在我帮您办理住院手续，请您稍等片刻。

N：Well, we're now at Interventional Therapy Department. My name is Xiao Na, you can call me Xiao Li.

I will help you with the admission procedure. Please wait for a moment.

患者：好的，谢谢。

P：OK，thank you.

护士：请问您的体重和身高分别是多少？

N：What is your weight and height?

患者：我身高 170 cm，体重 70 kg。

P：I am 170 cm and my weight is 70 kg.

护士：我需要询问您几个问题来完善您的病历。

N：I need to ask you a few questions to complete your medical record.

患者：可以。

P：Of course.

护士：请告诉我您的学历、职业及联系电话。

N：Please tell me your educational background，occupation and contact number.

患者：硕士学历，工作是经纪人，我的号码×××。

P：I have a master's degree，I am a broker and my number is ×××.

护士：请问您对什么药物过敏吗？比如青霉素？

N：Do you have drug allergies such as penicillin?

患者：没有。

P：No.

护士：请问您对什么食物、花粉过敏吗？

N：Are you allergic to any food or pollen?

患者：我现在还没有发现对任何东西过敏。

P：I don't think I have had any allergies so far.

护士：请问您有糖尿病、高血压等疾病吗？

N：Do you have diabetes，hypertension or any other diseases?

患者：没有。

P：No.

护士：最近您的食欲和睡眠如何？

N：How is your appetite and sleep?

患者：都还不错。

P：Not bad.

护士：您最近有没有哪里感觉不舒服或疼痛？

N：Do you feel uncomfortable or painful recently?

患者：暂时没有。

P：Not yet.

护士：好的，请您在这里签个字。我带您去床位，熟悉一下环境。

N：That's good，please sign here. I'll take you to your bed and show you around by the way.

患者：好的，谢谢。

P：OK，thank you.

护士：这里是医生办公室，刚刚那里是护士工作站，您有什么问题随时可以找我们。

N：This is the doctor's office. The nurse station is over there，you can turn to us whenever you need.

患者：谢谢。

P：Thank you.

护士：这里是厕所、洗澡间、洗漱间。那边有微波炉和24小时的热水供饮用。

N：Here is the toilet，bathroom and the washroom. Microwave oven is over there，and hot water for drinking is available for 24 hours.

患者：太好了。

P：That is great.

护士：这是您的床位，您是20床，这是呼叫铃，您需要帮助时可以打铃呼叫，我们会马上过来的。

N：This is your bed. Your bed number is 20. This is a bed alarm. You can ring the bell if you need any help，we'll come right away.

患者：好的。

P：OK.

护士：您还有什么想知道的吗？

N: Anything else you hope to know?

患者：没有了，我想到再问你，谢谢。

P: Nothing for now. I would ask you for help if anything comes to my mind. Thank you.

护士：您先休息一下，一会给您测个体温和血压。

N: Please have a rest for a while, and I will come to take your temperature and blood pressure later.

患者：好的。

P: No problem.

护士：谢谢您的配合。

N: Thanks for your cooperation.

[Phrases]

complete the medical record	完善病历
right away	马上
take the temperature	量体温
take the blood pressure	测血压

2. Health Education for Hospital Discharge
出院宣教

[Glossary]

discharge	出院
check out	结账
doctor's advice	医嘱
discharge certificate	出院证
deposit receipt	押金单
discharge summary	出院小结

[Scenario]

护士：刘先生，恭喜您明天可以康复出院了。

N：Mr. Liu，congratulations! You can be discharged from the hospital tomorrow.

患者：太好了，小李。

P：That's great，Xiao Li.

护士：根据医嘱，您明天就可以回家了。在出院前我还需给您交代一些注意事项。

N：According to the doctor's advice，you can go home tomorrow. I need to give you some discharge instructions before you leave.

患者：好的。

P：OK.

护士：您会结账吗？

N：Do you know how to check out?

患者：知道一点，不是特别清楚。

P：Only a little，I don't know the whole procedure.

护士：明天请记得带着出院证、出院小结、押金单和磁卡去5号楼1楼出院处结账。

N：All right，remember to bring your discharge certifi-

cate，discharge summary，deposit receipt and magnetic card to the discharge office on the 1st floor of
Building 5．

患者：这些单子在哪里？

P：Where can I get those documents?

护士：出院证和出院小结，医生会晚些给您，出院带药请结
账后在护士站领取。

N：The doctor will give you the discharge certificate and
discharge summary later，and you can get the medicine
from the nurse station after checking out.

患者：那我想复印病历呢？

P：What if I want to copy the medical records?

护士：您结完账，直接带着身份证去 3 号楼 4 楼病案室
复印。

N：You can take your ID card to the Record Room on the
4th floor of Building 3 after checking out.

患者：好的，我知道了。

P：OK，I got it.

护士：您回家后多注意休息，不要过度劳累。

N：Have more rest after getting home，and don't
overstress yourself.

患者：有什么东西不能吃的吗？

P：Is there anything that I can't eat?

护士：饮食上可以食用一些高蛋白、清淡、易消化的，多吃
些新鲜水果和蔬菜。回家如果有哪里不舒服，可以
打给护理站，电话是××××××××。

N：You can eat foods that are rich in protein，with mild
flavor and easy to digest. It is also beneficial to eat
more fresh fruits and vegetables. Just call us if you
don't feel well after getting home. The phone number
of our nurse station is ××××××××．

患者：好的，谢谢你。

P：OK，thank you.

护士：出院小结最后有口服药品的使用说明，请不要忘记。要按时按量，这样更利于尽快康复。

N：The instructions for oral drugs are listed at the end of the discharge summary, please don't forget that. Please take your medicine on time and in correct dosage so that you can recover as soon as possible.

患者：谢谢你的提醒。

P：Thank you for the information.

护士：请您在2个月后进行复查，检查项目在出院小结上，请您仔细阅读一下，有什么疑问可以问我。

N：Please remember to come for the checkup in 2 months. The required examinations are listed on the discharge summary. Please read it carefully. You can ask me if there are any questions.

患者：好的，我有问题再请教你。

P：OK，I will.

护士：请问您在住院期间对我们的护理还满意吗？

N：Are you satisfied with the nursing care during the hospitalization?

患者：谢谢小李在我住院期间对我的照顾，你们非常负责，谢谢。

P：Thank you for taking care of me，Xiao Li. All of you are very responsible，I do appreciate.

护士：谢谢您对我工作的肯定。一周后，我会给您打回访电话，有什么需要，可以告诉我，我会为你提供一些医疗帮助。

N：Thanks for your positive feedback. I will follow up and call you in a week. You can tell me what you want at that moment，and I will try to offer some help.

患者：好的，谢谢。

P：That's great，thank you.

护士：那您好好休息。

N：You're welcome. Have a good rest.

[**Phrases**]

be satisfied with	对……满意
during the hospitalization	住院期间
as soon as possible	尽快
be beneficial to	有益于

3. Fire Prevention Education
防火宣教

[Glossary]

detailed	详细的
evacuate	撤离
command	指挥
orderly	有序地
extinguish	熄灭
microwave	微波炉
continuously	持续地

[Scenario]

护士：陈阿姨，昨天我给您讲的防火知识还记得吗？

N：Ms. Chen, do you still remember the fire prevention tips that I told you yesterday?

患者：小高，我还记得，你讲得非常详细。

P：Yes, Xiao Gao, I still remember it, your guidance is very detailed.

护士：阿姨，那我考考您。

N：If so, I would like to ask you some questions to check.

患者：没问题。

P：No problem.

护士：如果发生火灾了怎么办？

N：What should you do if there is a fire?

患者：通知护士，然后撤离到安全的地方。

P：Inform the nurse and then evacuate to a safe place.

护士：怎么撤离呢？

N：How to evacuate?

患者：听护士的指挥有序撤离。

P：We shall follow the command of the nurse, and

evacuate from the ward orderly.

护士：嗯，那能不能坐电梯？

N：Well, can you take the elevator?

患者：不可以，要走两边的楼梯，而且要低位跋行，用湿毛巾堵住口鼻。

P：No, we should only evacuate from the stairs, and we should keep our body low, and use wet towels to cover our noses and mouths.

护士：如果自己身上起火，能不能奔跑？

N：If you happen to catch a fire on your body, can you run?

患者：不能，可以用水冲或就地打滚，直到熄灭身上的火。绝对不能带火逃跑，以免火势越来越大，增加伤害程度。

P：No, I may put out the fire with water or roll on the ground until the fire is extinguished. Never run with fire in order to prevent the fire from getting bigger and more harmful.

护士：怎么预防火灾？

N：How to prevent the fire?

患者：不能在病房里面吸烟或者使用明火，不能在微波炉转生食，这样时间长了，会短路，手机充电后要及时拔除，也不能使用高功率的电器，这些都是容易引发火灾的。

P：Do not smoke in the ward or use open flame. Do not heat up raw foods in the microwave, because it may cause a short circuit if the microwave works continuously for a long time. Unplug the phone when it is fully charged, and do not use high-power appliances, these can easily cause a fire.

护士：好的，看来宣教很有效。

N：All right. It seems that the fire education is effective.

[**Phrases**]

fire prevention	防火
safe place	安全地带
take the elevator	坐电梯
wet towel	湿毛巾
cover the nose	捂住鼻子
raw food	生食
short circuit	短路
high-power appliance	高功率电器

4. Burglary Prevention Education
防盗宣教

[Glossary]

burglary	盗窃
hospitalize	使……住院
remind	提醒
belonging	所有物

[Scenario]

护士：张先生，您是第一次住院吗？

N：Is this your first hospitalization，Mr. Zhang?

患者：是的，我以前没有住院治疗过。

P：Yes，I have never been hospitalized before.

护士：由于医院属于公共场所，有很多人在这里，所以您的贵重物品要保管好。

N：Because the hospital is a public place where there are a lot of people around，you should take care of your valuable belongings.

护士：我还需要特别提醒您，在离开病房时，随时带走自己的手机和钱包。夜间或者停电的时候是被盗高发时段，请特别注意一下。

N：I also need to remind you，please take your cell phone and wallet along with you when leaving the ward. Peak time of burglary is in the night or when power is off，please be precautious.

患者：嗯，谢谢提醒。

P：Well，thank you for reminding me.

护士：还有乘坐电梯时，请看管随身物品。

N：Please also take care of your belongings when you take the elevator.

患者：好的。

P：OK, I see.

护士：当然，一些不必要的贵重物品建议您在住院期间尽量放在家里，现在都是手机支付了，现金应该也不需要带那么多，有手机就可以了。

N：No doubt it is recommended that you put your valuable but dispensable items at home during your hospitalization, since mobile payment is popular now, it is not necessary to carry a lot of cash with you, you can do almost everything with just a phone.

患者：谢谢。

P：Thanks.

护士：不客气，有什么需要我做的，尽管找我，我叫高阳。

N：You're welcome. Please let me know whenever you are in need. My name is Gao Yang.

患者：好的，非常感谢。

P：OK, thank you very much.

[**Phrases**]

valuable belonging	贵重物品
it is recommended that ...	建议……
mobile payment	手机支付
peak time	高峰时段
take care of	看管

5. Fall Prevention Education
防跌倒坠床宣教

[Glossary]

cane	拐杖
urinal	尿壶
bedpan	便盆

[Scenario]

护士：李叔叔，今天是您住院的第一天，您还习惯吗？

N：Mr. Li, today is the first day of your stay in hospital. Are you getting used to it?

患者：我感觉很好，这里的医生、护士都很客气。

P：I feel fine. The doctors and nurses are nice here.

护士：您平时走路需要用拐杖或者需要别人帮助吗？

N：Do you usually walk with a cane or need help from others?

患者：不需要，我走路很稳。

P：No, I can walk relatively well.

护士：您躺在床上的时候最好将双侧床档全部拉起来，晚上睡觉的时候更加要注意，因为病床很小，翻身的时候可能会不小心掉下来。

N：When you on the bed, it is better to pull up both bed rails. At night you should pay more attention. Because the bed is narrow, you may fall off when you turn over.

患者：好的，我知道了。

P：All right, I see.

护士：还有，请把呼叫器放在容易拿到的地方。如果您家里人不在这里，您需要帮助的时候可以呼叫护士。

N：Also, you'd better put the bell within your reach. If

your family is not here, you can call the nurse when you need help.

患者：谢谢你。

P：Thank you very much.

护士：您如果需要上厕所，请不要将厕所的门从里面反锁，最好每次都有家属陪同。地面上如果有水的话，一定要小心，最好穿防滑拖鞋。晚上您也可以使用尿壶或者便盆。

N：If you need to go to the toilet, please don't lock the door from inside. It is better to have a family member with you every time you go to the toilet. If there is water on the ground, you must be careful. I suggest wearing antiskid slippers. At night, you can also use the urinal or the bedpan.

患者：好的。

P：Okay.

[Phrases]

turn over	翻身
go to the toilet	上厕所
antiskid slipper	防滑拖鞋

6. Smoking Cessation Education
戒烟宣教

[Glossary]

particle	颗粒
nicotine	尼古丁
monoxide	一氧化物
tar	焦油
ammonia	氨
benzene	苯
carcinogen	致癌物质
implement	实施

[Scenario]

护士：张爷爷，您好，我是您的责任护士小高。我可以问您几个问题吗？

N: Hello，Mr. Zhang. I'm your primary nurse Xiao Gao. May I ask you a few questions?

患者：当然可以。

P: Sure.

护士：请问您吸烟吗？烟龄大概是多少呢？

N: Do you smoke? If the answer is yes，how many years have you been smoking?

患者：是的，我吸烟大概 20 多年了。

P: Yes，about 20 years.

护士：那您知道吸烟有害健康吗？

N: Do you know that smoking is harmful to your health?

患者：我知道的。

P: Well，I know.

护士：目前全国每天有 2 000 余人死于吸烟，预计到 2050

年将增至 8 000 人。

N：More than 2 000 people die from smoking every day in our country，and this number is expected to increase to 8 000 by the year 2050.

患者：真是非常惊人的数字。

P：That number is really staggering.

护士：医学证实，每支烟燃烧时释放出 4 000 多种化学物质、几十亿个颗粒，含有尼古丁、一氧化碳、焦油、氨、苯等 69 种致癌物。

N：Medical research has shown that each cigarette releases more than 4 000 chemicals and billions of particles，which contain nicotine，carbon monoxide，tar，ammonia，benzene and other 69 carcinogens.

患者：听起来很可怕。

P：It sounds terrible.

护士：而二手烟对他人伤害更大。避免这种伤害唯一的办法就是戒烟。

N：And secondhand smoking is even more harmful to others. The only way to avoid this kind of injury is to quit smoking.

患者：我总是控制不住想吸烟，你有什么好的办法吗？

P：I just cannot control myself from smoking，do you have any good suggestions？

护士：首先，您得给自己树立能戒烟的信心。其次，给自己一些时间，您抽烟已经几十年了，想要戒烟并不容易。不抽烟时，您会出现一些不自觉的症状，如焦虑、口干、头疼等，这时需要转移注意，可以洗热水澡、多喝果汁、多做运动等。慢慢减少抽烟数量，这样您就会越抽越少，最后不想抽烟了。

N：First of all，you have to build up confidence. Then，give yourself some time. You have been smoking for decades and to quite it is not easy. You may have some unconscious symptoms when you stop smoking at the beginning. You need to divert your attention to other things if anxiety, dry mouth or headache occurs. For example, take a hot shower, drink fruit juice or do more exercises. You can reduce your cigarettes use, so that you will smoke less and less gradually, and eventually you may not want to smoke at all.

患者：真的有效吗？

P：Is it really effective?

护士：当然，只要肯坚持。您还需要学会拒绝他人给您的烟，告诉对方您正在戒烟。避免和喜欢抽烟的朋友待在密闭的环境中。

N：Of course, as long as you can keep doing it. You also need to learn to decline others' offering of cigarettes and tell them you are in cessation. Besides, try to avoid staying with friends who like smoking in the place without enough fresh air.

患者：我会尽我所能。

P：I will try my best.

护士：相信您一定能做到。病房里面不能吸烟您是知道的，如果真的很想抽烟的话，知道要去哪里吗？

N：I believe you will make it. You know that it is forbidden to smoke inside the ward, but if you really can't help it, do you know where to go?

患者：我知道的，楼下有专门的吸烟区域。从今天开始，我要慢慢戒烟，小高，你来督促我。

P：I know, there is a smoking area downstairs. Starting from today, I will reduce and quit smoking gradually, you are the supervisor, Xiao Gao.

护士：好的，张爷爷。

N：No problem, Mr. Zhang.

[**Phrases**]

quit smoking	戒烟
be harmful to	对……有害
be expected to	预计
increase to	增加到
secondhand smoking	二手烟
unconscious symptom	不自觉的症状
divert attention	转移注意力

7. Rest and Activity for Patients After Liver Cancer Surgery
肝癌患者术后的休息与活动

[Glossary]

appetite	胃口
proper	适当的
promote	促进
intestinal	肠道的
peristalsis	蠕动
defecation	排便
thrombosis	血栓
gastrointestinal	胃肠道的
pessimism	悲观主义
rupture	破裂

[Scenario]

护士：王伯伯，您在散步吗？

N：Mr. Wang, are you taking a walk?

患者：是的，小方。

P：Yes, Xiao Fang.

护士：今天感觉如何？较前两天有没有觉得舒服一些？

N：How are you today? Do you feel better than the last couple of days?

患者：前两天胃口不好，吃不下东西，脚上也没劲，今天好多了，所以下床多走了走。

P：My appetite was not very good in the last two days. I did not feel like eating anything. My feet were too weak to walk. But today I feel much better, so I get out of the bed and try to walk a little bit.

护士：非常好，您可以适当在床旁或病区内活动，以促进肠蠕动，早日排便，还可以增强食欲并预防深静脉血栓。

N：That's great. You can do some exercises at bedside or in the ward to promote intestinal peristalsis. It is also beneficial for defecation, and it can stimulate your appetite, and prevent deep vein thrombosis.

患者：是的，多活动，人也舒服很多。小方，我回家要注意什么？

P：Yes, more activities make me feel better. Xiao Fang, what should I pay attention to when I go home?

护士：适当体育锻炼可改善心、肺、胃肠道、神经系统功能，还可以消除悲观情绪。您回家以后，如果身体完全恢复了，可以适当做一些轻松的家务或一些体育锻炼，如散步、打太极拳等，但应以自己不感到疲劳为度。平时要避免用力、屏气等动作，以免因腹腔压力的变化导致肝癌破裂出血。

N：Proper physical exercises can not only improve the function of your heart, lung, gastrointestinal and nervous system, but also help you overcome pessimism. If you are in good condition, you can do some light housework or physical exercises like walking, tai-chi, and so on when you return home, but don't make yourself feel tired. Avoid exerting too much strength or holding breath, which may lead to sudden changes of intra-abdominal pressure, and cause rupture and bleeding of liver cancer.

患者：好的。

P：OK.

护士：如果遇到体温升高、有出血倾向、病情反复、白细胞低于正常值等情况，应停止锻炼，以免发生意外。

N：If you have a fever or bleeding tendency, or the

disease is refractory, or the white blood cell count is lower than normal, please stop exercising in order to avoid accidents.

患者：谢谢你的提醒。

P: Thank you for reminding me.

护士：除了适当的活动外，其实休息也很重要，每天要保持充足的睡眠，不要熬夜。

N: In addition to appropriate exercises, rest is also important. Please maintain an adequate sleep every day. Do not stay up late.

患者：我会的。

P: OK, I will.

[Phrases]

take a walk	散步
stimulate appetite	增加食欲
physical exercise	体育锻炼
nervous system	神经系统
light housework	轻松的家务
hold breath	屏气
intra-abdominal pressure	腹内压
bleeding tendency	出血倾向

8. Magnetic Resonance Imaging
磁共振成像

[Glossary]

MRI (magnetic resonance imaging)　　磁共振成像

pacemaker　　起搏器

enhanced　　增强的

suffocation　　窒息

[Scenario]

护士：王大志先生，您好，请让我看一下手腕带。

N：Hello, Mr. Wang Dazhi, may I see your wrist band?

患者：好的，在我的右手上。

P：OK, it's on my right hand.

护士：我是来给您通知明天的检查的。您明天中午12点要做一个肝脏的磁共振增强检查，现在我给您讲一下关于检查的注意事项。

N：I am here to inform you of the examination tomorrow. You will take an enhanced liver MRI examination at 12 o'clock tomorrow. Now I will give you some instructions about the examination.

患者：好的，护士。

P：OK.

护士：您有没有装过心脏起搏器等带有金属的植入物？

N：Do you have any metal implants? Like a pacemaker?

患者：没有，会有影响吗？

P：No, will it affect the examination?

护士：检查是不能携带含有金属的物件的，因为它们会与磁场发生反应。

N：Wearing metal objects are not allowed during the examination, as they will affect the magnetic field.

患者：哦，我有一颗金牙，还好能摘下来。

P：Oh，I have a gold tooth，but fortunately it can be taken off.

护士：那就好。因为您做的是增强，需要打造影剂，检查之前要禁食 4 个小时。极少数人会对造影剂过敏，出现呕吐等不适症状，这样在检查过程中非常容易引起窒息。

N：Good. You are going to do an enhanced MRI，therefore we will give you contrast medium. You can't eat anything 4 hours before the examination. Few people will have contrast agent allergies. In that case，vomiting and other symptoms may occur. Vomiting during the procedure may easily cause suffocation.

患者：好的，我晚上还能吃饭吗？

P：OK，can I eat at night?

护士：可以的，明天 8 点前都可以吃东西。

N：Yes，you can eat some foods by 8 o'clock tomorrow morning.

患者：好的。

P：OK.

护士：您不用太紧张，放松就好了。

N：You don't have to be too nervous. Take it easy.

患者：谢谢。

P：Thank you.

护士：不客气。如果有什么问题可以找我，我会给您解答的。

N：All right. Ring me for more questions you may have and I will be happy to answer.

患者：好的，谢谢护士。

P：OK，thank you.

[**Phrases**]

inform sb. of	通知某人……
metal implant	金属植入物
magnetic field	磁场
take off	取下
contrast agent	造影剂

9. Education for Patients Undergoing Gastroscopy
胃镜检查的健康教育

[Glossary]

gastroscope	胃镜
electronic	电子的
denture	假牙
anaesthetic	麻醉剂
throat	咽喉
mucosa	黏膜

[Scenario]

护士：您好，我是您的责任护士小迪。明天您要行电子胃镜检查，现在我给您讲解一下关于电子胃镜的注意事项。

N：Hello, I am your primary nurse Xiao Di. Tomorrow you will do an electronic gastroscopy. Now I would like to tell you some notes.

患者：好的。

P：OK.

护士：检查前需要禁食、水 6 个小时，确保空腹状态。如果您有活动性的假牙，也应先取出。

N：Don't eat or drink anything 6 hours before the examination to ensure an empty stomach. Active dentures should also be removed, if you have.

患者：做胃镜疼吗？

P：Will I feel pain during gastroscopy?

护士：检查前会适当地给您使用麻醉剂的，不用太担心。检查后，短时间内因为麻醉的作用，您的咽喉部可能会有异物感，不要用力咳嗽，以免损伤黏膜。

N：The doctor will give you some anaesthetics before the examination, so don't worry too much. Your throat may feel uncomfortable for a short period of time after the examination due to the effect of anaethetic. Please do not cough forcefully to avoid mucosa damage.

患者：好的,那我做完检查之后什么时候可以进食呢?

P：I see. When can I eat after the examination?

护士：检查后,如果您的咽喉麻醉作用尚未完全消退,不能立即进食,1～2 小时后可饮水,如无呛咳可进食。1 天内进清淡少渣的饮食,3 天内避免进刺激性的食物,以免引起黏膜出血,同时也应注意观察大便的颜色及有无腹痛等症状。如有不适,请及时告知我们。

N：You should not eat before the effect of anaethetic disappears after the examination. Usually you can drink water 1 to 2 hours later and resume eating if you don't cough. On the first day you can eat some light and low-residue foods. Please avoid eating irritative foods in 3 days to avoid mucosal bleeding. At the same time, pay attention to observing the color of your stool and whether you have abdominal pain. Please inform me in time if you don't feel fine.

患者：好的,护士。谢谢你的宣教。

P：OK. Thank you for your information.

护士：不用谢,那您好好休息。如果有什么事情,请按铃呼叫我,我也会经常来看您的。

N：You are welcome, have a good rest. If you need any help, ring the bell please, I will also check on you regularly.

患者：好的。

P：OK.

[**Phrases**]

a short period of time	短时间
mucosal bleeding	黏膜出血
abdominal pain	腹痛

10. Education for Patients Undergoing Colonoscopy
　　肠镜检查的健康教育

[Glossary]

colonoscopy	肠镜检查
fast	禁食
magnesium	镁
sulfate	硫酸盐
nausea	恶心
defecation	排便
polypectomy	息肉切除
rehydration	补液

[Scenario]

护士：苏先生，您好，我是您的责任护士小迪。您的肠镜检查约到了，在后天早上 8 点。

N：Hello, Mr. Su. I'm your primary nurse Xiao Di. Your colonoscopy is scheduled at 8 a. m. the day after tomorrow.

患者：怎么要等三天？我希望明天就做肠镜检查。

P：Why do I have to wait for three days? I hope to have it done tomorrow.

护士：不要着急，检查前您需要做一些准备工作，让肠镜检查更加顺利，现在我来给您讲一下注意事项。

N：Don't worry. Before the examination, it is necessary for you to get prepared so that your colonoscopy can be carried out more smoothly. I am now going to give you the instructions for colonoscopy.

患者：好的。

P：OK.

护士：肠镜检查前三天需控制饮食：第一天是半流质、少渣
　　　饮食；第二天是流质；最后一天需要禁食。

N：Please start to control your diets 3 days before the
　　examination：semifluid and low-residue diets 3 days
　　before the test；liquid diets 2 days before the test；do
　　not eat the day before the test.

患者：好的，谢谢护士。那我检查前需要准备些什么呢？

P：All right，thank you. Is there anything that I need to
　　do before the check？

护士：在检查前 4～5 小时，50 克硫酸镁粉加温开水 100 ml
　　　口服，也可将硫酸镁混入饮料后口服，然后缓慢饮用
　　　白开水，以不感到明显腹胀为标准。此后 1 小时内
　　　口服温开水 2 000～2 500 ml。服药后会出现腹泻，
　　　我们会观察您大便的情况，直到大便为清水样无粪
　　　渣才可做肠镜检查。如果出现恶心、呕吐等不适症
　　　状，需告诉我们，我们会给您清洁灌肠的。

N：You need to take orally 50 g of magnesium sulfate
　　powder with 100 ml warm water 4 to 5 hours before
　　the check，or mix it with a drink，then slowly drink
　　some warm water as long as you don't feel bloated.
　　After that，drink 2 000～2 500 ml warm water in 1
　　hour. You will have diarrhea for several times after
　　taking the medicine. We will keep observing your
　　stool. Only when it appears clearly watery with no
　　fecal residue can you do the colonoscopy. If you have
　　nausea，vomiting and other symptoms，just tell us，we
　　will give you an cleansing enema.

患者：一般排几次才能干净？

P：How many times does it normally take to make my
　　bowel empty？

护士：一般半小时左右开始排便，连泻 5～7 次即可基本排
　　　清大肠内粪便。

N：Defecation begins in about half an hour, and you'll need 5～7 times to fully evacuate the feces inside your bowel.

患者：如果我在检查过程中疼痛难忍怎么办？

P：What should I do if I feel pain during the check?

护士：如果您在检查过程中腹痛难忍，请及时告诉操作医生，医生会给您处理的。

N：If you can't tolerate the abdominal pain during the examination, please inform the operating doctor immediately and the doctor will handle the situation in time.

患者：那我做完检查后什么时候可以吃东西呢？

P：When can I eat after the examination?

护士：做完肠镜后如无不适，2 小时后可进食。饮食也要根据医嘱来定。有活组织病理检查或息肉摘除治疗的，当天晚上禁食，根据您的情况，给予补液治疗。检查后可能有少量的大便带血，一般情况不须特殊处理，但如果出血较多，请及时告知我们，我们会给您处理的。

N：You can eat 2 hours after the colonoscopy if you don't have any discomfort. Your diets should also be based on the doctor's advice. If biopsy or polypectomy is required, you will have to fast at night. According to your situation, we will give you a rehydration treatment. After the examination, mild blood stool may occur. It does not need special treatment in general. But if the symptom is severe, please inform us promptly, and we will deal with it in time.

患者：好的，谢谢护士！

P：Got it, thank you!

护士：不用谢，那您好好休息。

N：My pleasure, have a good rest.

[**Phrases**]

the day after tomorrow	后天
semifluid	半流质
liquid diet	流质饮食
warm water	温开水
be based on	基于……

11. Official Account Promotion
公众号推广

[Glossary]

WeChat	微信
rehabilitation	康复
registration	注册
assistant	助手
input	输入
nutrition	营养
repository	知识库

[Scenario]

患者：小李，你们的康复助手我怎么登不进去？

P：Xiao Li, I can't log in the Rehabilitation Assistant.

护士：让我来看看，您是用微信登录的吗？

N：Let me see. Did you log in with WeChat?

患者：是的。

P：Yes.

护士：您需要先搜索微信公众号中的康复助手，然后关注它，并扫描我们的二维码，您要的信息就会出现了。

N：Search WeChat for Rehabilitation Assistant, subscribe to it, and then scan our QR code. The information you want will be shown.

患者：你能帮我一下吗？

P：Could you give me a hand?

护士：当然！您看"发现"这里，有"扫一扫"，或者输入课程码，您要看什么内容？

N：Sure. Just click "Discover" and you will find "Scan", or you can also input the course code. What are you going to read?

患者：我想看肝癌介入治疗。

P：I'd like to read the information about interventional therapy for liver cancer.

护士：点"今日"进入肝癌介入手术康复指导界面。输入入院时间后，您就可以收到系统发送的信息提醒。它涉及的范围有疾病、护理、手术、康复、营养、出院、检查等，您自己也可以随时查询。

N：OK, click "Today", you will be navigated to the rehabilitation guidance interface for liver cancer interventional surgery. By inputting the admission time, you will receive the message sent by the system. It includes disease information，nursing, operation，rehabilitation，nutrition，discharge，examination，etc. You can always search for them as long as you want to.

患者：你们的内容很丰富！怎么还有营养？

P：So many contents! I can see that the nutrition is also included.

护士：是的，这是康复助手的知识库，它会经常推送科普知识，帮助患者建立健康的饮食习惯。

N：Yes，this is the repository of Rehabilitation Assistant. It will often send popular science knowledge and help our patients to build up a healthy diet habit.

患者：这个很好啊！自从我患病后，家里人很多东西就不让我吃了，我要好好看看才行。

P：This is very good! After I got ill, my family doesn't allow me to eat a lot of things. I will read it carefully.

护士：对的，其实正确的饮食能预防很多疾病，也能治好很多疾病，您要充满信心才行。

N：In fact, a proper diet can help you prevent and even cure many diseases. You should be confident.

患者：谢谢你的鼓励。

P: Thanks for your encouragement.

护士: 我们医院也有微信公众号, 我帮您也加一下, 这样下次挂号就不用等了, 直接网上预约, 可以节约时间, 里面还可以查询费用和血检查报告等。

N: We also have our own WeChat official account. Let me help you make the subscription. Next time you can directly make an appointment on the net instead of waiting for registration, which will save you a lot of time. You can also use it to check your medical expense and blood test report.

患者: 那太好了!

P: That is really good!

[**Phrases**]

official account	公众号
QR code	二维码
interventional therapy	介入治疗
rehabilitation guidance	康复指导
diet habit	饮食习惯
make an appointment	预约